# CORONARY ARTERY DISEASE

## Advances in Detection & Treatment

### 2019 Report

A Special Report published by
the editors of *Heart Advisor*
in cooperation with Cleveland Clinic

*Coronary Artery Disease: Advances in Detection & Treatment*

Consulting Editor: Leslie Cho, MD, Director, Women's Cardiovascular Center; Co-Section Head, Preventive Cardiology and Rehabilitation, Robert and Suzanne Tomsich Department of Cardiovascular Medicine, Cleveland Clinic

Author: Holly Strawbridge
Creative Director, Belvoir Media Group: Judi Crouse
Editor, Belvoir Media Group: Jay Roland
Production: Mary Francis McGavic

Publisher, Belvoir Media Group: Timothy H. Cole
Executive Editor, Book Division, Belvoir Media Group: Lynn Russo Whylly

ISBN 978-1-879620-79-7

To order additional copies of this report or for customer service questions, please call 877-300-0253, or write to Health Special Reports, 535 Connecticut Avenue, Norwalk, CT 06854-1713.

This publication is intended to provide readers with accurate and timely medical news and information. It is not intended to give personal medical advice, which should be obtained directly from a physician. We regret that we cannot respond to individual inquiries about personal health matters.

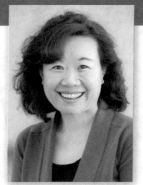

**Leslie Cho MD, FACC, FSCAI, FESC**
Professor of Medicine, Cleveland Clinic Lerner School of Medicine Case Western Reserve Medical School Director, Women's Cardiovascular Center and Co-Section Head, Preventive Cardiology and Rehabilitation

**C**oronary artery disease (CAD) causes more deaths in the U.S. than all forms of cancer combined. That's because CAD is the reason for heart attack, an event about 805,000 men and women in the U.S. experience each year and 114,00 die from. CAD is also the most common form of cardiovascular disease—a condition that causes stroke, kidney failure, and poor blood flow to the legs and feet that often requires amputation.

The good news is that the death rate from CAD has been falling steadily. Many doctors, including my colleagues here at Cleveland Clinic, are developing new interventions and medications to save lives. We are learning how CAD behaves differently in women than in men. We're learning more about treatments that can help people live longer after being diagnosed with heart disease. And very importantly, more people like you are adopting heart-healthy behaviors to manage their CAD or prevent heart disease from developing in the first place. That means eating a better diet, exercising more, and following your doctor's instructions on medications, quitting smoking, controlling your weight, getting regular checkups, and more.

Reading this report is yet another heart-healthy choice. You'll learn how the heart works and how CAD develops. You'll also learn what you can do to lower your odds of developing CAD, and how you can make the best decisions if you're already dealing with heart disease. We've compiled some of the latest studies and treatment guidelines to help you stay up-to-date with how cardiologists, heart surgeons, and researchers are taking on this dreaded disease.

CAD remains a major health threat, but reading this report is an important step in giving you and your loved ones your best chances of surviving and thriving long into the future.

Wishing you and your family good health and a long life,

Sincerely,

*leslie Cho*

Leslie Cho MD, FACC, FSCAI, FESC

# TABLE OF CONTENTS

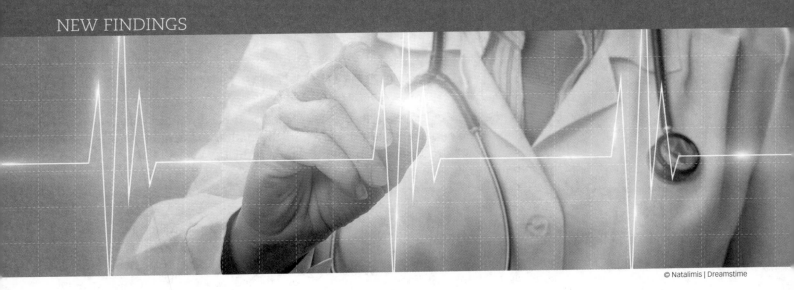

© Natalimis | Dreamstime

# Report on Coronary Artery Disease

New medicines, devices, and procedures to help manage heart disease and prevent heart attacks and heart failure have dramatically changed the prognosis for patients with coronary artery disease (CAD). Between 2003 and 2015, the number of deaths from CAD dropped 28 percent, primarily due to lowering cholesterol, controlling blood pressure, and quitting smoking. Despite this good news, around 14 percent of people who experience a heart attack in any given year die from it.

Your ability to survive and thrive with CAD is influenced somewhat by where you live. A 2016 study found that people living in the Deep South had the highest mortality rates from heart disease, followed by those in the southern Appalachians. This was a dramatic change from 40 years earlier, when mortality rates from heart disease were highest in the Northeastern United States.

The more you know about CAD, how to prevent it from progressing, and how it is treated at different stages, the more likely you will be to keep consequences of the disease at bay. In this report, you will learn how your doctor will determine the severity of your disease, what drugs you will need to take, and what lifestyle changes you may need to make to help your heart stay healthy. You will learn what procedures are available to restore blood flow to your heart and what you can do to help prevent a heart attack. By learning how to manage your disease and get the best treatment, you'll have the best chance of restoring your heart to good health.

## About Cleveland Clinic

The Cleveland Clinic's Sydell and Arnold Miller Family Heart & Vascular Institute is the largest and busiest heart center in America. **It has been recognized as No. 1 in the nation for cardiology and heart surgery in** *U.S. News & World Report's* **"America's Best Hospitals" issue every year since 1994.** Cleveland Clinic specialists have made breakthroughs that helped to define modern cardiac care—coronary angiography, coronary artery bypass surgery, minimally invasive valve procedures, and refined robotic techniques, to name but a few—and continue to innovate for better outcomes and experience. With an international reputation for excellence, Cleveland Clinic welcomes patients from around the nation and throughout the world.

Cleveland Clinic services are provided through a unique model of medicine. Here are some of the factors that set it apart:

- **Every physician is a salaried employee.** All Cleveland Clinic physicians are salaried to ensure that patient care, not financial gain, remains their top priority. This practice eliminates incentives to perform unnecessary tests or procedures and encourages physicians to consult with colleagues and spend the time necessary to practice excellent medicine.
- **Care is delivered through integrated practice units called institutes.** Each institute combines medical and surgical departments related to the management of one organ system or disease area into a single organizational entity under a single leadership team. The Miller Family Heart & Vascular Institute combines cardiovascular medicine, thoracic and cardiovascular surgery, vascular surgery and all their subspecialties into one unit outfitted with the most advanced medical and surgical equipment.
- **Nurses and physicians collaborate closely on patient care.** Cleveland Clinic nurses are recognized and respected for the key role they play in patient care and

## Facilities for State-of-the-Art Care

The Sydell and Arnold Miller Family Pavilion, a 1 million-square-foot, state-of-the-art center opened in 2008, is dedicated exclusively to heart and vascular care. The facility includes such features as a robotic surgery suite, 12 catheterization labs, 16 spacious operating rooms, seven fully equipped electrophysiology labs, and 278 private patient rooms. Cutting-edge cardiac radiology and nuclear medicine services are provided on site, and the center includes a 21-bed dialysis suite, as well as a rooftop helipad to receive critically ill or injured patients. The facility comprises dedicated intensive care units for heart failure, coronary care, and cardiovascular and thoracic surgery, with a total of 110 beds.

The Miller Family Heart & Vascular Institute at Cleveland Clinic, home of the country's largest cardiovascular practice, employs more than 227 physicians who provide care for more than 600,000 outpatient visits and 13,000 hospital admissions. They perform more than 4,500 cardiac surgeries a year, which includes more than 1,500 coronary artery bypass graftings and 3,000 valve operations, plus more than 1,800 lung operations and 2,700 vascular surgeries. Patients come from more than 80 countries and all 50 states.

are encouraged to speak up when they note a problem or have concerns.

- **Cleveland Clinic encourages research.** In fact, so much research is performed at Cleveland Clinic that the physicians and nurses are able to identify promising technologies early and begin using them. Cleveland Clinic's cardiovascular team has kept meticulous computerized records of procedures and outcomes since 1971, building an unmatched outcomes database. The data is used to fuel research and to continuously refine treatment approaches.

- **Innovation is valued.** Physicians are both permitted and encouraged to "think outside the box" to find better ways of treating heart disease. The culture of innovation not only results in developing new devices and treatments, but also in new ways of delivering care and improving the coordination of care.

- **Education is fully supported.** Cleveland Clinic pays for physicians to spend time elsewhere to learn new procedures or techniques.

- **Cleveland Clinic uses advanced health information technology,** including electronic medical records (EMRs). EMRs enable physicians to spend more time with patients and less time doing paperwork, and make care safer by having instant access to patients' records at all times. By using state-of-the-art technology-based systems that are true medical tools, Cleveland Clinic is able to meet its physicians' needs and better serve patients.

- **Every patient death is documented and reviewed.** In an institution that accepts some of the sickest heart patients in the world, this practice creates a learning environment that helps keep mortality rates among the lowest in the nation.

- **Ultimately,** Cleveland Clinic strives to put patients first by treating all patients, as well as colleagues, as if they were close family members.

## A History of Innovation

### Selected Discoveries and Advances

- Breakthroughs in understanding high blood pressure and its links to heart disease
- Pioneering open-heart surgery on a stopped heart
- Discovery of the enzyme angiotensin and its role in high blood pressure
- Development of implantable artificial hearts
- Discovery of coronary angiography
- Discovery of the first gene associated with familial heart attacks
- Creation of a test for myeloperoxidase, a biomarker for heart attack
- Discovery of the role of gut flora-dependent TMAO in atherosclerosis and other cardiometabolic diseases and a medication that prevents the gut from making TMAO

### Selected Innovations and Firsts

- First coronary artery bypass surgery
- First dedicated cardiothoracic anesthesiology department
- First heart transplant in Ohio
- First heart/double-lung transplant in Ohio
- First heart-liver transplant in Ohio
- First minimally invasive mitral valve operation in the world
- First computerized database for cardiovascular diagnosis and treatment
- Development of tissue-lined stent to treat peripheral vascular disease
- Invention of a clip device to exclude the left atrial appendage and prevent stroke in patients with atrial fibrillation

### Development of an annuloplasty ring for valve repair

- Invention of a closure device for repairing septal defects
- Invention of a wire-free breastbone-closure device that speeds healing and eliminates slippage

### Selected Therapies and Procedures

- Pioneering work with arterial bypass grafts in cardiac surgery to increase survival rates
- Development of blood-conservation techniques to eliminate the need for transfusion in many patients
- Development of new valve-repair techniques
- Introduction of intravenous thrombolytic (clot-busting) therapy for heart attacks
- Use of intravascular ultrasound (IVUS) to visualize plaque in artery walls
- Pioneering of surgical treatment for atrial fibrillation
- Development of a debris catcher to improve the safety of carotid stenting

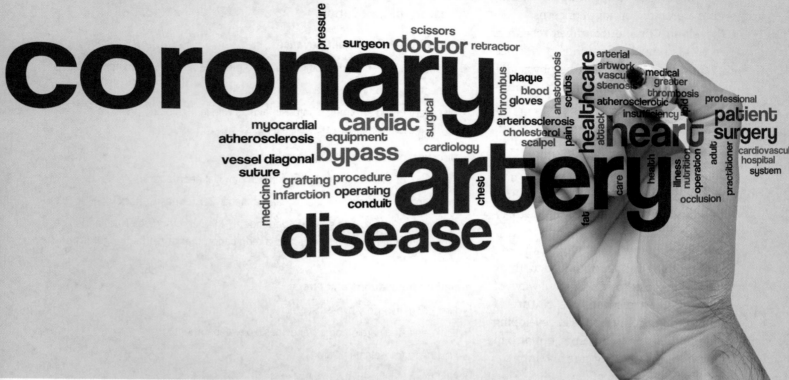

© ibreakstock | Dreamstime

Coronary artery disease (CAD) is a major health problem in the U.S., but improvements in prevention and treatment are saving lives.

# 1 Cardiac Care Is Advancing Rapidly

Coronary artery disease (CAD) is a disease that limits or blocks blood flow in the arteries that supply blood to the heart muscle. CAD is caused by atherosclerosis, a process in which cholesterol, fats, and white blood cells accumulate inside the walls of coronary arteries, forming plaques. Soft, young plaques are more likely than older, stable plaques to rupture and release their contents into the bloodstream. This triggers the body to release enzymes that cause blood to clot. Stable plaques form through a slower process that occurs over time. The arteries can become narrowed by hard, calcium-rich plaques until blood flow is seriously impaired. No matter the cause, a blockage in a coronary artery leads to a heart attack. Blood flow stops and the heart muscle cannot contract normally. If blood flow is not restored quickly, heart muscle tissue dies. It is possible to recover from a

small heart attack, but damage to a large amount of heart tissue can kill you.

At least three processes that cause atherosclerosis are known. The first is turbulent blood flow at the junction where two arteries meet. In this case, extreme force on the blood vessel wall may injure the vessel and enable cholesterol molecules, as well as other molecules called reactive oxygen species, to take hold and impair vascular function.

The second process is the reaction of the body's immune system to atherosclerotic plaques. Blood vessels tend to view plaques as foreign bodies and recruit white blood cells to attack the invaders. These cells release more potentially damaging reactive oxygen species. They also can explode after taking in too much cholesterol, starting the harmful cycle all over again.

The third process is remodeling. Once the blood vessels have grown as large as

## How Coronary Artery Disease Develops and a Heart Attack Happens

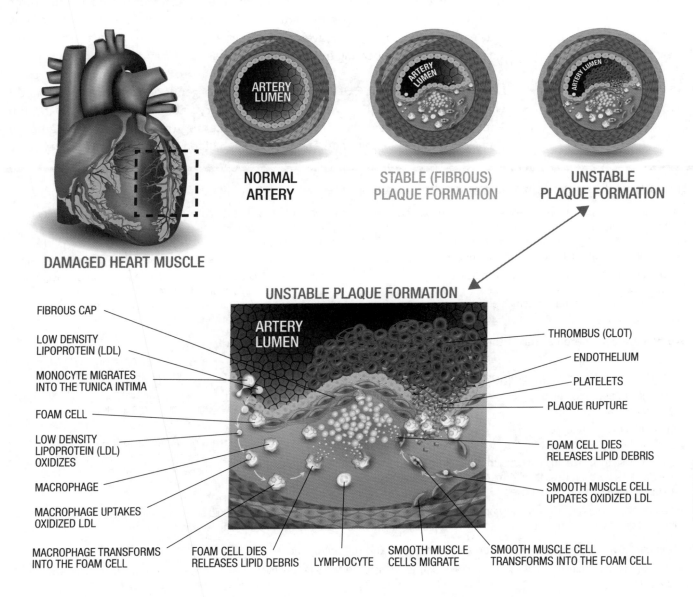

DAMAGED HEART MUSCLE

NORMAL ARTERY

STABLE (FIBROUS) PLAQUE FORMATION

UNSTABLE PLAQUE FORMATION

### UNSTABLE PLAQUE FORMATION

ARTERY LUMEN

FIBROUS CAP

LOW DENSITY LIPOPROTEIN (LDL)

MONOCYTE MIGRATES INTO THE TUNICA INTIMA

FOAM CELL

LOW DENSITY LIPOPROTEIN (LDL) OXIDIZES

MACROPHAGE

MACROPHAGE UPTAKES OXIDIZED LDL

MACROPHAGE TRANSFORMS INTO THE FOAM CELL

FOAM CELL DIES RELEASES LIPID DEBRIS

LYMPHOCYTE

SMOOTH MUSCLE CELLS MIGRATE

SMOOTH MUSCLE CELL TRANSFORMS INTO THE FOAM CELL

THROMBUS (CLOT)

ENDOTHELIUM

PLATELETS

PLAQUE RUPTURE

FOAM CELL DIES RELEASES LIPID DEBRIS

SMOOTH MUSCLE CELL UPDATES OXIDIZED LDL

© Guniita | Dreamstime

A normal artery has three layers. The first layer on the inside of the artery is the intima. It comes in direct contact with flowing blood. The intima consists of a layer of specialized endothelial cells (endothelium) that are in direct contact with the blood. The endothelium lies on a matrix consisting of fibrous proteins. Underneath the intima is the media, a layer composed mainly of muscle cells that can contract and relax (dilate) to regulate the flow of blood through the artery. The media also contains fibrous and elastic proteins that provide support and enable the artery to stretch without breaking. The layer on the outside of the artery is called the adventitia. This layer of fibrous proteins contains nerves to stimulate contraction and relaxation of the smooth muscle cells in the media.

In atherosclerosis, injury to the endothelium stimulates a healing response similar to inflammation. But as a result of the injury, cholesterol and other fats (lipids) are deposited in the intima. If the cause of the injury is removed, the endothelium will be restored to normal.

If the injury is repetitive, this abnormal deposit grows and becomes a plaque. White blood cells and other types of cells begin to migrate into the intima in an attempt to remove or isolate the plaque. Platelets also stick to the injured endothelium, becoming incorporated into the plaque along with small blood clots. This phase is called maturation. As described in the text, some plaques are stable while others are vulnerable. Vulnerable plaques are prone to rupture, stimulating the formation of a blood clot.

If the blood clot becomes large enough to completely block what remains of the artery's lumen, blood will stop flowing through the artery, causing a heart attack.

possible, their walls grow inward, restricting blood flow.

Fortunately, ongoing efforts to identify CAD earlier, treat it more effectively, and, ideally, prevent it, are bearing fruit.

## Differences Between Men and Women

There are biological differences in the way CAD manifests in women and men. In women, the disease tends to affect the smaller arteries in the heart, and often affects arteries in other parts of the body, as well. In men, CAD tends to affect larger vessels. The way plaques grow, rupture, and lead to heart attacks is the same in both genders. Yet heart attack is the primary cause of heart failure in men, weakening the heart's pumping power. High blood pressure is the primary cause

### How Women Can Prevent Heart and Cardiovascular Disease

American Heart Association guidelines for preventing and managing cardiovascular disease in women assign women to one of three tiers: high risk, at risk, or having ideal cardiovascular health (the optimal and lowest level of risk).

Those in the highest risk stratum are not difficult to identify because they have known symptomatic cardiovascular disease or high-risk features such as abdominal aortic aneurysm, end-stage kidney disease, diabetes, or a calculated

10-year risk of cardiovascular events greater than 10 percent. Their optimal treatment has been verified in multiple large-scale clinical trials.

The "at risk" category is a different matter entirely, since identifying these individuals is not always straightforward. This group represents the lion's share of the female population, probably amounting to more than 70 percent of women between the ages of 50 and 79 years.

**Women are considered at risk if they have one or more of the following major risk factors:**

- Ongoing tobacco use
- Family history of cardiovascular disease
- Evidence of asymptomatic atherosclerosis
- Untreated blood pressure greater than 120/80 mmHg
- Total cholesterol greater than or equal to 200 mg/dL, HDL-cholesterol less than 50 mg/dL, or treatment for abnormal lipid levels

- Poor diet
- Metabolic syndrome
- Obesity (body mass index [BMI] greater than 30 kg/m2), particularly with the "apple" body shape
- Physical inactivity
- Poor performance on an exercise treadmill test

- A systemic autoimmune disease, such as lupus or rheumatoid arthritis
- History of preeclampsia, gestational diabetes, or pregnancy-induced hypertension.
- More recently, early onset hot flashes (between ages 40 and 53) have been identified as a risk factor for CAD.

Given its expansive definition, many women will wind up in the "at risk" category. Doctors should seek to identify these women and initiate aggressive preventive cardiovascular therapies. The goal is to move them into the next-lower risk category.

**Ideal cardiovascular health is defined as having all of the following characteristics:**

- Untreated total cholesterol level less than 200 mg/dL
- Untreated blood pressure less than 120/80 mmHg

- Untreated fasting blood glucose level less than 100 mg/dL
- Body mass index (BMI) less than 25 kg/m2
- Abstinence from smoking

- Meeting recommended levels of physical activity
- Following a diet similar to the one used in the Dietary Approaches to Stop Hypertension (DASH) trial.

**Some key points of the guidelines include:**

- Accumulate at least 150 minutes of moderate exercise or 75 minutes of vigorous exercise per week, with sustained aerobic activity for at least 10 minutes per episode, and perform strengthening exercises involving all major muscle groups at least two days a week.

- Follow a daily diet that includes more than 4.5 cups of fruits and vegetables, 30 grams of fiber, three servings of whole grains, and four servings of nuts. Also, the diet should contain less than one tablespoon of sugar, one teaspoon of salt or the equivalent of 2,300 mg per day (1,500 mg if you have high blood pressure). and 150 mg of cholesterol. Less than seven percent of total calories should come from saturated fats.

- Consume 1,800 mg per day of omega-3 fatty acids in fish or capsule form. This is especially advisable for women with high cholesterol, high triglycerides, or both.

- Avoid therapies without proven benefit or with risks that may outweigh benefit, such as noncontraceptive hormone therapy without indications for symptomatic relief, antioxidant vitamin supplements, and routine use of aspirin in healthy women under age 65.

- Complete guidelines can be found on www.goredforwomen.org/about-heart-disease/heart-disease-news/new-heart-disease-prevention-guidelines/.

of heart failure in women, making the heart stiff.

There are differences in the timing and severity of CAD, too. Men tend to have heart attacks at a younger age than women. Men are also at a higher risk than women for developing CAD at some point in their lives.

In addition, there are situations specific to women that increase the risk of CAD. These include having gestational diabetes, gestational high blood pressure, and poly- cystic ovary disease. In 2016, endometriosis was found to raise the risk of developing CAD by 62 percent: In women aged 40 and younger, endometriosis increased the risk by a frightening 400 percent! More recently, frequent hot flashes between the ages of 40 and 53 were identified as a risk factor. Sadly, radiation therapy for breast cancer and cer- tain chemotherapy agents used in treating the disease increase the risk of developing heart failure, even without CAD.

Physicians have only recently become aware of significant gender differences in many risk factors for CAD, including lip- ids, biomarkers of inflammation, endo- thelial dysfunction, stress and injury to heart-muscle cells (myocytes), and kidney function. Therefore, men and women may be better served with different diagnostic tests. In some cases, different treatments may be needed to achieve the best results. But there is good news: Mortality from car- diovascular disease has decreased more than 33 percent in women over the last 15 years, likely due to better recognition and management of CAD before a heart attack occurs.

## Identifying New Populations at Risk

Atherosclerosis can occur in arteries throughout the body. That's why people with coronary artery disease also may have plaques in their brain (cerebrovascu- lar disease), kidneys (renal disease), legs and feet (peripheral artery disease, or PAD), and other places. Studies have found such a strong association between heart attack and stroke in people with PAD that some physicians now call PAD an independent risk factor for heart attack. Other research has shown that the risk of stroke increases after a heart attack, and vice versa.

The systemic nature of cardiovascular disease also can cause erectile dysfunc- tion (ED) in men. Although ED is not fatal, it can interfere with quality of life. In many cases, ED serves as an important early warning sign of CAD or diabetes. The good news is that sildenafil (Viagra), a common drug used to treat ED, dilates blood ves- sels and, in the process, lowers blood pres- sure, increases circulation, and protects the heart and lungs from stress.

## The Importance of Individualized Treatment

CAD is not a simple disease. Many factors are involved in raising the risk in any given person. The risk is always relative, meaning there is no way to say that if you take cer- tain steps, you will not get CAD, or your CAD will disappear. However, there are known risk factors for CAD that, if treated, will lower the risk.

There is no "one-size-fits-all" treatment. Instead, individualized treatment plans work best. These plans take into account a person's age, cholesterol levels, co-existing diseases such as diabetes or hypertension, lifestyle habits such as smoking, the pres- ence of certain proteins in the blood, and, increasingly, gender. With a growing num- ber of options for treating heart disease, information obtained from a wide variety of tests, combined with knowledge about what works in similar patients, is helping doctors make more informed decisions about which treatments to recommend for each patient.

## Better Non-Surgical Treatments

Treatment for CAD can include medica- tion, coronary artery bypass grafting (CABG, which means bypass surgery), or an inter- ventional procedure, such as angioplasty with stenting. In CABG, a piece of artery

## Coronary Artery Bypass Surgery

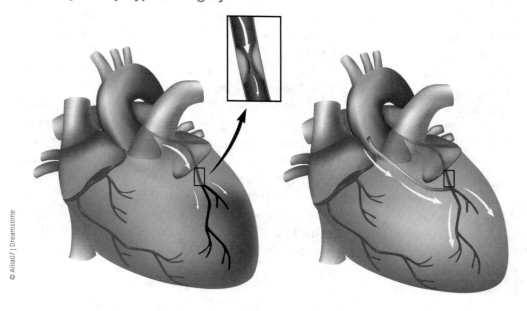

In coronary artery bypass surgery, a heart surgeon takes a vein or artery (or arteries) from another part of the body and sews it onto a coronary artery that has become blocked. Blood flow is rerouted through the grafted blood vessel, thus bypassing the blockage.

from the chest wall or a vein from the leg is grafted onto a narrowed artery to reroute blood around the blockage.

Rather than bypassing blocked coronary arteries, many patients undergo a percutaneous coronary intervention such as angioplasty and stenting. In this procedure, plaque is pushed out of the way with a little balloon inflated at the site of the blockage. A tiny mesh tube called a stent is then inserted into the diseased coronary artery to prevent it from collapsing. Stents may have bare metal surfaces or be coated with a drug to prevent scar tissue from growing inside the stent and re-narrowing the opening ("in-stent restenosis").

The procedure that is right for you depends on where the disease is located in your arteries and how much disease is present. This topic is discussed in greater detail in Chapter 6.

The fact is that more than one treatment is often needed to prevent a heart attack, slow the progression of CAD, and delay the need for a repeat procedure. Today, patients who do not require surgery usually take several medications. When a surgical or an interventional procedure is necessary, medications can improve success rates and long-term survival. The addition of counseling, extended follow-up with a health-care provider, and careful attention to diet and exercise provide the most effective ways to reduce heart disease.

### Less-Invasive and "Off-Pump" Bypass Surgery

A CABG procedure that could be performed without opening the chest, but rather by going through small openings between the ribs, was immediately embraced. In this procedure, the surgeon controls a robotic arm to perform the most delicate operations on the heart. Because a heart-lung machine is not required to breathe for the patient, the technique can be used on many patients for whom traditional heart surgery would pose a serious risk, including those with liver disease or a diseased ascending aorta.

The popularity of off-pump surgery peaked in 2002 and has declined since.

Various clinical studies have reached conflicting conclusions as to its safety. Likewise, minimally invasive robotic CABG has its benefits and risks. The current advice is to reserve these procedures for appropriate patients, rather than making them the default operations.

## Standardizing Care

During a heart attack, giving certain medications within a specific time frame improves the chance of recovery. Hospitals and emergency medical personnel throughout the country now utilize accepted protocols for treating heart attack. This means patients in rural hospitals are likely to be treated the same way as those at urban medical centers. New protocols sometimes require heart attack patients to be stabilized and transferred to a hospital with more sophisticated facilities to ensure they receive the best care.

## Proven Prevention

We have learned that certain risk factors for coronary artery disease can be modified through diet, dietary supplements, medications, exercise, and lifestyle change. These will be explained in more detail in Chapter 3.

The value of healthy eating and regular exercise in preventing a heart attack is well known. Research also has shown that some protective benefits can be derived from meditation to lower stress.

High cholesterol levels can be lowered through the use of medications called statins. There is even evidence that statins may protect against early mortality, whether or not you have heart disease.

Another way to prevent heart disease is to get a full physical checkup. Although this may seem obvious, there is a significant lack of awareness about individual risk, particularly among young women. This is a troubling fact, considering that heart disease is the No. 1 killer of U.S. women, and the rate of heart disease deaths in women ages 35 to 44 continues to climb every year.

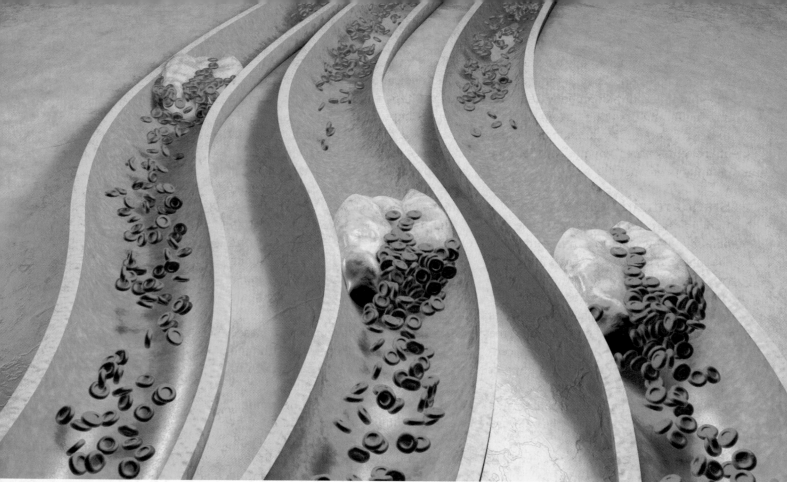

The symptoms of CAD can appear suddenly, but the buildup of plaque in the coronary arteries can take decades to accumulate.

## 2 How Coronary Artery Disease Occurs

Your heart pumps about 2,000 gallons of blood every day. When it's working fine, you probably don't give it much thought. However, if your heart develops a problem such as CAD, you'll begin to appreciate every beat.

CAD takes a long time to form. Plaque development starts at an early age and continues over many years. Most people don't know they have coronary artery disease until about 70 percent of the inside of an artery (the lumen) becomes blocked. At this point, they may experience chest pain known as angina.

In a normal artery, healthy endothelial cells lining the inside of the artery provide a smooth surface for blood to flow across and help prevent blood from clotting unnecessarily. In the early stages of plaque development, the endothelial cells begin to change in response to repetitive exposure to stresses or toxic substances, such as cigarette smoke, air pollution, diabetes, high blood pressure, or high cholesterol.

Injured endothelial cells interact with the white blood cells flowing past them. White blood cells are programmed to carry away cells and tissues that are killed or damaged to pave the way for the growth of new cells and tissues. In an injured coronary artery, white blood cells arrive in great numbers to help repair the damage. Instead of flowing past, they stick to the endothelial cells and crawl between them to get inside the wall of the artery, where they accumulate. This results in inflammation.

If the risk factor injuring the endothelial cells is removed—say, by quitting smoking, or lowering high blood pressure or high cholesterol—the endothelial cells can heal. But if the injury keeps happening, white blood cells continue to be recruited. Plaques develop from a combination of these white blood cells and lipids such as cholesterol. These plaques form streaks in the artery wall.

## Chronology of Clotting

When plaques reach a certain size, five things begin to happen:

- White blood cells inside the fatty streak begin to die and release cholesterol, forming what is known as the necrotic (dead) core of the plaque.
- Smooth muscle cells in the arterial wall begin to multiply to cover the necrotic core.
- Blood cells called platelets, which are essential to clotting, begin to stick to the injured endothelial cells, and help form small blood clots on the surface of the necrotic core.
- Platelets and blood cells begin to mix with the muscle cells covering the necrotic core to form a fibrous cap.

### What Is Cholesterol?

Cholesterol is a type of lipid (fat-soluble molecule) made in the liver and obtained from food. The body requires only a small amount of cholesterol to make hormones, bile, and vitamin D. Extra cholesterol may be deposited on artery walls throughout the body. Because lipids do not mix with water, cholesterol hitches a ride through the bloodstream by piggybacking on proteins. The combinations are tiny spheres called lipoproteins. There are four main types of lipoproteins, but patients with CAD should be concerned mainly with low-density lipoproteins (LDL) and high-density lipoproteins (HDL). The cholesterol carried by LDL can be deposited in the arteries, which increases the risk of heart disease and stroke. Thus, LDL is considered "bad" cholesterol. Conversely, cholesterol carried by HDL is transported from arteries to the liver for removal from the body, so it is considered "good" cholesterol.

### The Heart—A Pump We Take for Granted

The heart—revered as the source of romantic feelings—is really just a pump. In healthy people at rest, the heart beats between 60 and 100 times every minute. Exercise, emotional stress, and certain hormones can cause it to beat faster.

Special cells in the heart generate electrical impulses that stimulate the muscle to squeeze rhythmically (the systole phase). This allows the heart's lower chambers, the ventricles, to send the blood coursing through the body or directly to the lungs for oxygenation. Between beats, the heart relaxes and fills with blood for the next beat (the diastole phase).

Blood flow to the heart muscle fuels this process. Blood is supplied by two main arteries on the heart's surface. The right coronary artery supplies the right ventricle, which pumps blood to the lungs, as well as the back of the left ventricle, which pumps blood to the body.

The left coronary artery, which is about the width of a soda straw, supplies a larger share of the left ventricle's muscle. This coronary artery divides into the left anterior descending coronary artery, which runs down the front of the heart and supplies blood to the tip (apex) of the heart muscle, and the left circumflex artery, which circles around and feeds the left side of the heart.

Oxygenated blood
Unoxygenated blood

Ascending aorta (to upper body)

Aorta (to body)

Superior vena cava (from upper body)

Left pulmonary artery (to left lung)

Right pulmonary artery (to right lung)

Left atrium

Right pulmonary veins (from right lung)

Left pulmonary veins (from left lung)

Right atrium

AV

MV

PV

Inferior vena cava (from lower body)

Left ventricle

TV

Right ventricle

AV = Aortic valve
MV = Mitral valve
PV = Pulmonary valve
TV = Tricuspid valve

Decending aorta (to lower body)

© Allia07 | Dreamstime

Each artery divides into smaller and smaller branches until they become so small that red blood cells flow through them in single file. These smallest vessels are called capillaries, and it is here that the heart muscle exchanges its carbon dioxide and metabolic waste for oxygen and nutrients.

Blood returns to the heart through a network of veins that empty the blood directly into the right atrium, one of the heart's upper chambers.

• Cells in the developing plaque begin to deposit calcium inside the plaque, making it hard.

In addition to impeding blood flow, plaques affect the ability of arteries to dilate and contract, which is necessary to adjust blood flow to the demands of tissues and organs. This is called the elastic property of arteries, and it is what you feel as your pulse. Because plaques are hard to the touch and change the artery from a flexible, soft tube to a rigid pipe, the growth of plaques was previously called "hardening of the arteries."

Until plaques become complex and mature, they have virtually no effect on blood flow or the dilation and contraction of coronary arteries. At this point, CAD is asymptomatic. It's only when the plaques begin to restrict the amount of blood passing through a coronary artery that you become aware of CAD's first symptom— usually a type of chest discomfort called angina. Angina is a sign of ischemia (pronounced *iss-KEE-mee-uh),* or insufficient blood supply to the heart.

Plaques with thin walls can rupture easily, often without warning. These so-called "vulnerable plaques" are difficult to identify, because they often do not contain calcium or narrow the interior diameter of the artery (lumen). Therefore, they tend to elude detection by angiography or stress tests. Finding a way to identify these vulnerable plaques is a priority, but to date no reliable way to detect them has been found.

Stable plaques have a smaller fatty core and more supporting structures, which are readily visible on angiography.

## Elevated Risks

Whether your plaques are vulnerable or stable, you are at increased risk for heart attack. Oddly, plaque is not disrupted in about one-third of patients with unstable angina, heart attack, or sudden cardiac death. That means there was no apparent stimulus for their blood to clot. It turns out that certain risk factors—including high levels of "bad" cholesterol, the toxins in cigarette smoke, and high blood sugar levels—make blood more "clottable." Chronic inflammation increases blood levels of certain proteins and other factors, producing the same effect. As a result, plaque doesn't always need to rupture to cause a blood clot that results in unstable angina or a heart attack.

The fat surrounding the outside of arteries—particularly the right coronary artery—also may influence the onset of coronary artery disease. This outer fat, known as perivascular fat tissue, is different from fat found beneath the skin in other parts of the body (see "Amount of Perivascular Fat May Reveal Risk of Death"). Perivascular fat tissue in people with coronary artery disease is highly inflamed, and there is growing evidence it may be a culprit in the formation of fatty plaques.

## Stable Angina

Patients describe angina in various ways, as a "heaviness" or "pressure" in the chest or a tight "squeezing" or "smothering" sensation. Whatever the description, it is usually frightening enough to cause the person to seek medical help. Angina is often triggered by exertion or powerful emotions that make the heart race, increasing its demand for oxygen and nutrients. When

**NEW FINDING**

### Amount of Perivascular Fat May Reveal Risk of Death

A novel biomarker that focuses on fat around the coronary arteries has been found to predict death from CAD and other causes better than any other method. The biomarker, known as the fat attenuation index (FAI), was developed after researchers found that inflammation in the coronary arteries inhibits new fat from forming in surrounding tissue. The FAI enables physicians to measure inflammation-induced changes in existing fat using CT angiography. The results reveal patients at risk from small plaques that are highly inflamed and unstable.

To develop and test the FAI, researchers at Cleveland Clinic and a German hospital collected data from nearly 4,000 patients undergoing coronary CT angiography and mapped the fat surrounding their three major coronary arteries. They discovered that changes in the fat around the left anterior descending artery and, in particular, the proximal right artery strongly predicted the risk of death within a median of five or six years. Because half of all heart attacks occur in patients with no evidence of atherosclerosis on coronary angiography, this technique may make it possible to identify those who are at risk and intervene before a heart attack occurs.

*Lancet,* Sept. 15, 2018

plaques prevent an adequate supply of oxygen-rich blood from getting through, chest pain occurs.

If the episodes are relatively short, predictable with respect to time of day, amount of exertion and emotional state, and relieved by rest, you probably have chronic, stable angina. If your doctor confirms this diagnosis and recommends medical treatment or lifestyle changes, it is in your best interest to follow the advice rigorously to minimize the risk of developing unstable angina or having a heart attack. Heart attacks occur in 20 percent of people with this kind of predictable, stable angina.

Once you are diagnosed with chronic stable angina, treatment will focus on diminishing the severity and frequency of your episodes of angina. The overall goal is to avoid progression to unstable angina and heart attack.

## Unstable Angina

In many patients, angina becomes severe and/or occurs three or more times per day. It may occur with little exertion, or be almost constant, occurring even at rest. This is unstable angina, and it requires immediate medical attention.

Unstable angina is much more serious than stable angina, because it may be caused by a plaque in the process of rupturing. When a small rupture occurs, a small blood clot may briefly stop blood flow before the body dissolves it. This causes the chest discomfort. When blood flow is restored, the angina is relieved until the next little blood clot forms. The danger is that the blood clot will stick and grow, stopping blood flow long enough to cause a heart attack. That's why emergency medical care is necessary.

Unstable angina puts you at extremely high risk for a heart attack. You should be admitted to the hospital to stabilize your condition and avoid a heart attack. More than likely you will need stenting or CABG.

Although it's tempting to think elderly adults might be too fragile for invasive treatment, this is not true. In a 2016 study, adults over age 80 did better when treated with stenting or CABG plus optimal medical therapy than they did with medications alone. At 1½ years after the initial incident, 40.6 percent of patients who had undergone invasive treatment and 61.4 percent of those receiving medical treatment had suffered a heart attack or stroke, needed urgent revascularization, or had died. However, after age 90, the advantages of the invasive strategy were "diluted."

After undergoing stenting or CABG, you will need to make lifestyle modifications and take medications to lower your risk of another episode of unstable angina or heart attack.

## Heart Attack

In unstable angina, the heart muscle is starved for oxygen and nutrients, but it recovers quickly when blood flow is restored. That's not always the case when you have a heart attack.

Heart attacks can happen in people who have no clue they have CAD, because they did not have symptoms. The severity of a heart attack is generally determined by how much heart muscle is affected and how long the blood flow is stopped. This is why it is necessary to seek emergency care immediately if you suspect you are having a heart attack. Because the symptoms of a heart attack are many, and can be different in women than in men, it is wise to learn them. In others, there is no chance for a quick restoration of blood flow, and they die.

Heart attacks can sometimes cause an abnormal heart rhythm called ventricular fibrillation (VF), which is usually fatal without immediate treatment. A heart in VF quivers and cannot pump blood. As a result, the person usually collapses and experiences what is known as sudden cardiac death. Rhythm often can be restored by shocking the heart with an external defibrillator. Automated external defibrillators (AEDs) are kept in

## Anatomy of a Heart Attack

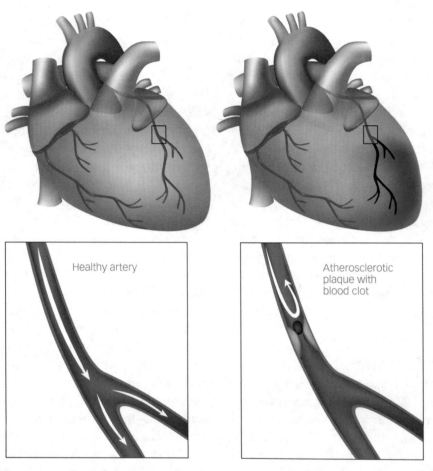

When plaque—made up of cholesterol, fats and other materials—forms in the walls of a coronary artery, the stage is set for a heart attack. If the plaque ruptures, a blood clot can form quickly in the artery, blocking blood flow through the artery and starving the heart muscle of oxygen. This injury to heart tissue is called a heart attack. Restoring blood flow as quickly as possible is the key to successful heart attack treatment.

many public places, including airports and shopping malls. A normal heart rhythm must be restored within a couple of minutes, or irreparable brain damage will occur. Until the patient regains a pulse, cardiopulmonary resuscitation (CPR) must be done to keep oxygen-carrying blood flowing to vital organs. In the event that an AED cannot be used, the American Heart Association recommends doing chest compressions (cardiopulmonary resuscitation, or CPR) until an ambulance arrives.

The immediate goal of treatment is to limit damage by relieving the blockage either medically or surgically. The likelihood of surviving without complications and resuming a normal lifestyle depends on how long your heart muscle has been subjected to insufficient blood flow, and how much of your heart is permanently damaged.

Once you have had a heart attack, you are up to 15 times more likely to have a second heart attack, stroke, angina, heart failure, or die from sudden cardiac arrest. This is why you should also eliminate or treat any risk factors that still may apply to you, through lifestyle modifications and medical therapy.

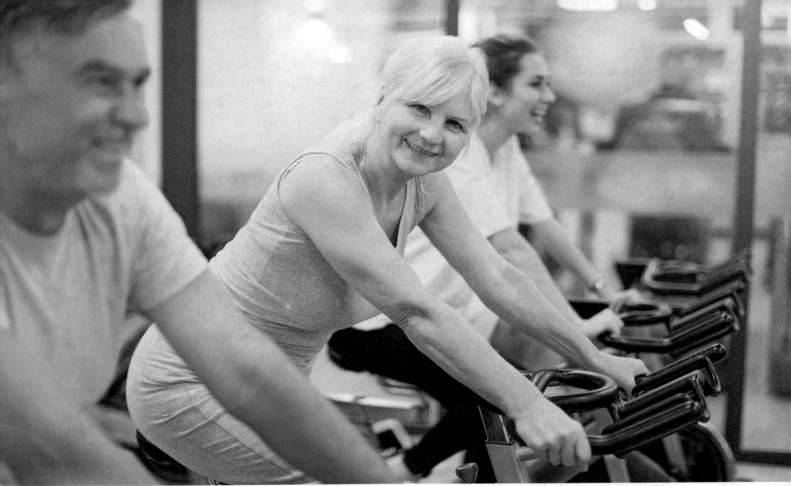

A lifestyle characterized by regular exercise and a heart-healthy diet can help lower the risk of CAD and its many complications.

# 3 Lowering the Risk of CAD and Heart Attack

Many risk factors for CAD are well established, and new factors are coming to light. The presence of any one risk factor increases the risk of heart disease, and multiple risk factors increase the risk exponentially. Because the risk of CAD increases with age, you may have CAD, even if you don't have any conventional risk factors (see "No Cardiovascular Risk Factors? You May Still Have Atherosclerosis" on page 20). If you have any risk factor for heart attack, plaques are growing in your coronary arteries. Unfortunately, there is no accepted way to confirm this with testing. Despite the promotion of resting or stress electrocardiography, stress echocardiography, or stress myocardial perfusion imaging tests for screening purposes, these tests have not been shown to improve outcomes. In fact, the high rate of false positive results increases the risk of undergoing cardiac catheterization needlessly.

It is possible, however, to reduce the risk of heart attack through lifestyle modification or medical treatment, making it wiser to treat risk factors than to wait for symptoms to appear. The advice for preventing a first heart attack is the same as for preventing a second one, but there are exceptions (see "Aspirin No Longer Recommended for Primary Prevention" on page 21).

You can begin to improve your health by starting and maintaining healthy habits with help from the American Heart Association's healthy living initiatives: *Go Red for Women*. These resources provide simple solutions for improving nutrition, physical activity, and children's health. For more information, visit www.americanheart.org.

Two-thirds of people with diabetes die from heart disease or stroke. However, a survey conducted by the American Diabetes Association found that 68 percent of people with diabetes do not consider cardiovascular disease to be a serious complication of their diabetes.

—*American Diabetes Association*

## No Cardiovascular Risk Factors? You May Still Have Atherosclerosis

Although the presence of atherosclerosis is closely tied to conventional cardiovascular risk factors, freedom from these risk factors does not necessarily mean freedom from atherosclerosis. A study of nearly 1,800 middle-aged nonsmokers with optimal or normal blood pressure, blood sugar, and blood lipid levels found that 50 percent had atherosclerosis, and 30 percent had the disease in multiple vessels. The highest risk of atherosclerosis was associated with older age, male sex and high LDL-cholesterol levels. LDL was the strongest modifiable risk factor associated with atherosclerosis, even when all other risk factors were optimal. This suggests LDL levels should be much lower than are currently recommended.

*Journal of the American College of Cardiology,* Dec. 19, 2017

## Certain Risk Factors Prove Worse for Women than Men

High blood pressure, diabetes, and smoking are known to increase the risk of heart disease. Now a study of nearly 500,000 adults—more than half of them female—found these traditional risk factors have a worse impact on women than on men.

In women, the risk conferred by high blood pressure was 80 percent higher than in men. The risk from type 1 diabetes was three times higher and from type 2 diabetes was 47 percent higher. Smoking doubled the risk in men, but tripled it in women.

The George Institute for Global Health Nov. 7, 2018

The good news is that the steps to prevent CAD are the same steps that can reduce your risk of heart attack, once you have been diagnosed with CAD. If you have CAD, however, lifestyle modifications alone are not likely to reduce your risk to an acceptable level. Combining lifestyle modifications with medical, interventional cardiac, or surgical therapy are much more effective than any single therapy alone.

## Types of Risk Factors

Risk factors can be divided into two categories: non-modifiable (not changeable) and modifiable (changeable).

## Non-Modifiable Risk Factors

### Family History

CAD tends to run in families, as do other conditions that are risk factors for CAD, including diabetes, high cholesterol, and high blood pressure. If your father or brother had heart disease before age 55, or your mother or sister had it before age 65, then your risk is especially high. Women with a genetic risk may have a heart attack in their 20s, 30s, or 40s. Fortunately, even if a CAD risk factor like high blood pressure runs in your family, you may be able to reduce your risk with lifestyle modifications and moderate exercise.

### Age

Your risk of developing CAD and having a heart attack increases with age. If you suffer a heart attack at age 75, you are twice as likely to die from it than if you have a heart attack at 65. Women are at much less risk than men until they reach menopause, after which their risk increases greatly.

### Gender

Men and women are at equal risk of having coronary artery disease. However, a man is 2½ times more likely to die from heart disease in his 40s than a woman. The average age for a first heart attack is 65 in men, 70 in women. After menopause, when the protective effects of estrogen disappear, the rate of heart attack in women skyrockets and quickly equals that of men. Women who undergo menopause early are twice as likely to suffer from CAD, regardless of ethnicity or other traditional cardiovascular disease risk factors. The negative impact of early menopause is similar whether a woman reaches it naturally or through surgical removal of her reproductive organs in a hysterectomy. However, a woman is more likely than a man to die from her first heart attack. Unfortunately, efforts to stave off heart disease with estrogen replacement therapy do not work.

### Race

Heart disease is the leading cause of death in people of all races. However, blacks are more likely than whites to die from their heart disease, while Hispanics, East Asians, and Native Americans are less likely to have a heart attack than whites. South Asians have a particularly high risk of heart attack.

## Modifiable Risk Factors

Obviously, you can't grow younger or modify your genes, but you can lower additional risk from modifiable risk factors. (See Certain Risk Factors Prove Worse for Women than Men.) If you are elderly, are of a race or gender that carries a higher risk, and/or have a family history of heart disease, it's even more important that you attempt to reduce or eliminate any modifiable risk factors that apply to you. These include:

### Smoking

Smokers are two to three times more likely than nonsmokers to develop CAD, and they develop the disease about 10 years earlier. Smokers also are two to four times more likely to die suddenly from a heart attack. Research also shows that stroke survivors who smoke are at a greater risk for a heart attack. The good news is that quitting smoking, but not cutting down on the number of cigarettes you smoke, can reduce the risk of heart attack or stroke, even if you quit after age 60 (see "Cutting Back on Cigarettes Doesn't Work, on page 21").

## Abnormal Cholesterol and/or Triglyceride Levels

Cholesterol and triglycerides are fat-soluble substances necessary for normal cellular functions. Excess amounts, however, contribute to the development of atherosclerosis. Higher blood levels of low-density lipoprotein (LDL) cholesterol or triglycerides and lower levels of high-density lipoprotein (HDL) cholesterol have been linked to an increased risk of developing CAD and having a heart attack or developing aortic valve disease. Since the development of atherosclerosis is a gradual process, everyone should have a cholesterol check at age 20 and every five years thereafter. If you have a family history of heart disease, you should have a full cholesterol profile test yearly starting at age 20 to delineate levels of total cholesterol, LDL, HDL, and triglycerides.

## High Blood Pressure

It's called "the silent killer" for good reason: People with high blood pressure (hypertension) may not know they have it, but uncontrolled hypertension more than doubles the risk of heart attack. According to the American Heart Association, hypertension (blood pressure higher than 130/80 mmHg) is found in 51 percent of people with CAD, 69 percent of people who have a first heart attack, 77 percent of people who have a first stroke, and 74 percent of people with heart failure.

## Diabetes

Patients with type 2 (adult-onset) diabetes are generally overweight and have high blood pressure and cholesterol. Diabetes doubles or triples the risk of a heart attack.

## Obesity

If you are 20 percent or more over the recommended weight on a standard height-weight table, you are considered obese. Your heart must strain to pump blood through miles of extra vessels, and you are twice as likely to have high blood pressure and diabetes. The higher your body mass index (BMI), the greater your risk of heart attack at a younger age.

## Physical Inactivity

People who don't exercise have almost twice the risk of heart attack. Exercise strengthens the heart muscle, lowers blood pressure and cholesterol, and helps control weight.

## Environment

No matter what climate you live in, you are more likely to die of heart-related issues during the winter. Researchers hypothesize that the colder temperatures might increase blood vessel constriction and raise blood pressure. It's recommended that you maintain healthy habits, such as eating a balanced diet and exercising regularly, during the winter months and year 'round. Moreover, research has found that heat waves and cold spells lasting two or more days can lead to premature death from heart attack, likely by triggering changes in blood pressure, blood thickness, cholesterol, and heart rate.

A clean environment helps to protect your heart, as well. Air pollution, especially in the form of particulate matter, can damage your heart. You would be wise to avoid vehicle exhaust and smoke created by burning wood or waste products.

## Other Risk Factors

Other risk factors that could be important include endometriosis, low estrogen levels occurring in menopause, low testosterone levels, the amount of specific proteins in your blood, previous treatment for certain cancers, and diseases such as pneumonia. (This is why you should check with your doctor about whether an annual pneumonia vaccine is right for you.)

Psychological stresses, such as depression and loneliness, can worsen heart health, as well. This may explain why middle-aged and older dog owners were found to be less likely to die from

NEW FINDING

### Aspirin No Longer Recommended for Primary Prevention

It used to be thought that low-dose aspirin could prevent a first heart attack, but recent clinical trials have found the risks to be far greater than the benefits for most people. In ASCEND, daily aspirin in patients with diabetes resulted in a modest 12 percent reduction in CV events, but a 29 percent increase in major internal bleeding. In ARRIVE, which involved patients without diabetes at moderate CV risk, daily aspirin had no effect on death or heart attack, but increased the risk of gastrointestinal bleeding. In ASPREE, a study involving adults ages 70 and older, aspirin had no effect on the composite outcome of death, dementia, and disability. When these outcomes were taken alone, the rate of deaths, primarily due to cancer, was higher in those taking aspirin than placebo. What does this mean for you? The decision to take daily aspirin should be made on an individual basis after careful consultation with your physician.

*New England Journal of Medicine*, online Aug. 26, 2018; *Lancet*, online Aug. 26, 2018; *New England Journal of Medicine*, online Sept. 16, 2018

NEW FINDING

### Cutting Back on Cigarettes Doesn't Work

If you think that only a couple cigarettes a day won't hurt, a meta-analysis of 141 prospective studies found you are wrong. Many people think they are doing their health a favor by cutting their smoking from a pack or more a day to a couple of cigarettes. The researchers expected to verify the benefits of this practice. Instead, they discovered that smoking only one cigarette a day increases your cardiovascular risk about 50 percent if you're a man and 75 percent if you're a woman. The only way to reduce the excess cardiovascular risk is to quit smoking completely.

*BMJ*, online Jan. 25, 2018

cardiovascular disease than their peers who didn't own dogs: The companionship a dog provides that decreases loneliness may be responsible. (The exercise gained from daily dog walking may help reduce weight and blood pressure, as well.)

Although certain bacteria are sometimes found in plaques, antibiotic therapy has failed to make any impact on plaque or on the occurrence of heart attacks. This finding suggests that bacterial infection is not a cause of CAD.

## Assessing Your Risk

The message is clear: quit smoking, get regular exercise, lose weight, lower your cholesterol, control your blood pressure, and, if you have diabetes, watch your blood sugar. You may get sick and tired of hearing this advice, but the fact is that if you take it to heart, you will lower your chance of developing CAD. If you already have CAD, controlling these risk factors will reduce your chance of having a first or second heart attack.

Even small changes—for example, cutting back on sugar—can make a big impact. The American Heart Association recommends limiting added sugar (sugar not naturally occurring in fruit and fruit juice) to 100 calories a day for women and 150 calories a day for men.

Although these measures have been proven to lower risk, 25 to 50 percent of people who follow them will still develop

CAD. Physicians have long suspected that other risk factors are involved, and several have now been identified. Some are genetic in origin, and some are caused by inflammation. The different factors that increase the risk of a heart attack confirm that the development of CAD is a complex process.

The solutions are not simple. Everyone is unique, and the factors that cause one person to develop CAD may be different from those influencing the disease process in another. That's why it's necessary to identify the individual factors that influence your risk.

## Modifying the Risk Factors You Can

Whether you have CAD or seek to prevent it, consider each modifiable risk factor that applies to you as an opportunity to take control. After all, you have only one heart. You would be wise to protect it.

### Smoking

Although any amount of smoking raises the risk of a heart attack, risk increases in proportion to the number of cigarettes you smoke. People who smoke two or more packs of cigarettes a day are at least three times as likely to develop CAD as nonsmokers. Those who smoke a pack a day have more than twice the risk. The longer you smoke, the greater your risk will be. Even "part-time" smoking is dangerous.

Women who smoke—even those without a history of heart disease or stroke—have nearly 2½ times the risk of sudden cardiac death, compared with healthy women who do not smoke. For every five years of continued smoking, the risk climbs by 8 percent.

The good news is that the risk of a heart attack actually begins to decrease after you smoke your last cigarette. Of all the modifiable risk factors, quitting smoking has the greatest effect on lowering risk. When you quit smoking, your risk will drop by 50 percent over the next two to four years. However, you will remain at increased risk for 10 years or longer.

NEW FINDING

**Safety of Smoking-Cessation Drugs Confirmed**

Many people find nicotine replacement products and medications to be helpful for quitting smoking. Yet concerns that they may have caused heart attacks has persisted. These fears prompted the FDA and its European counterpart to conduct a double-blind, randomized, triple-dummy, placebo- and active-controlled trial involving more than 8,000 adult smokers in multiple countries. All received at least one dose of varenicline (Chantix®, Champix®) or buproprion (Wellbutrin®, Zyban®) or a nicotine patch. More than half were treated for 12 weeks, then followed for an additional 40 weeks. At the end of the study period, few cardiac events had occurred. No significant differences were found in the blood pressure, heart rate, or time to cardiovascular event in the treatment groups, or between the treatment and placebo groups. The researchers concluded there was no evidence that smoking-cessation therapies increase the risk of serious cardiovascular events during or after treatment, at least for typical smokers at no elevated risk for heart disease.
*JAMA Internal Medicine,* April 9, 2018

There's no question that quitting is hard, but millions of people do it every year. You are twice as likely to be successful if you use a nicotine-replacement product, such as a nicotine patch, gum, nasal spray, or inhaler. Two smoking-cessation drugs are now available: bupropion and varenicline. Each drug works differently, and research shows you will be more successful if you utilize three stop-smoking aids simultaneously (see "Safety of Smoking-Cessation Drugs Confirmed").

It is also important to avoid areas where people smoke, because exposure to secondhand smoke has been shown to increase the risk of developing CAD by 30 percent. The adverse health effects of passive smoke are thought to be virtually as dangerous as active smoking. You have plenty of company if you've tried before and failed, but don't give up. Your chance of success gets better with each subsequent attempt. Don't get discouraged: Most smokers try to quit five to seven times before they finally succeed.

With increasing frequency, people are turning to other products to break their tobacco habit. These may not be better choices.

E-cigarettes typically contain nicotine, in addition to a flavoring agent and a solvent. As with tobacco cigarettes, the nicotine is addicting. Additionally, while the flavoring agents are safe to eat, their safety when inhaled in unknown. Some vaping liquids also contain undesirable products such as anabasine, which is principally used as an insecticide.

Marijuana is another tobacco substitute growing in popularity as it becomes decriminalized. However, its safety for people with, or at risk for heart disease, is unknown (see "Marijuana's Effect on the Heart Remains Uncertain").

## Abnormal Cholesterol and/ or Triglyceride Levels

Cholesterol and fats are necessary for life. We get them from the foods we eat. Triglycerides, another type of fat, are the body's main energy storage molecules and are stored in fat tissue. Although many people have become aware of the dangers of high "bad" cholesterol levels, they may be less familiar with triglycerides. The increasing prevalence of obesity and diabetes in our country is likely responsible for these elevated triglyceride levels.

Triglyceride and cholesterol molecules are wrapped in tiny, protein-covered spheres that move easily through the bloodstream. These particles are called lipoproteins. Low-density lipoproteins (LDL) and high-density lipoproteins (HDL)

**NEW FINDING**

### Marijuana's Effect on the Heart Remains Uncertain

Do we know how safe marijuana is? Recent research suggests we do not.

A group of researchers collected all studies of marijuana published in English between January 1975 and September 2017. There were only 24, and only one was well designed. It was a 3,882-patient case-crossover study that looked at marijuana as a potential trigger of heart attack and found increased risk in the first hour after smoking marijuana. The other studies had too few participants, or were too poorly constructed, to draw conclusions.

Another study was more concerning. It concluded that regular marijuana use may triple the risk of death from hypertension. In this study of 1,213 people who had ever smoked marijuana or cigarettes, marijuana users had a risk of death from hypertension that was 3.42 times higher than nonusers, even when study participants diagnosed with hypertension were excluded from the calculation. The association between current and former cigarette smokers and death from hypertension was much lower.

*Annals of Internal Medicine,* online Jan. 23, 2018; *European Journal of Preventive Cardiology,* Aug. 8, 2017

## Tips for Quitting Smoking

- **Be committed.** Acknowledge that quitting smoking is a difficult undertaking that requires a lot of effort.

- **Discuss smoking-cessation programs** and nicotine-replacement therapy with your doctor. Using three approaches simultaneously— for example, a prescription smoking-cessation drug, the nicotine patch, and nicotine gum— will increase your chance of success.

- **Mobilize a support team.** Ask your family, friends, and coworkers to support your efforts.

- **Be goal-oriented.** Set a definite date to be "smoke-free," rather than simply trying to cut back.

- **Use mental imagery** to imagine yourself as a successful non-smoker.

- **Give yourself positive feedback.** When you crave a cigarette, tell yourself, "I can handle it," or, "It will go away soon." Then find a substitute—drink some water, eat a piece of hard candy, get a sponge and squeeze it repeatedly, start doodling, call a friend on the telephone, take a deep breath—anything to distract your mouth and hands.

- **Don't focus on possible weight gain.** The few pounds you might add are far less of a health risk than smoking.

- **Don't try to diet at the same time.** It will hinder your success.

## Hypertension

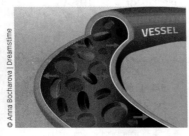

Blood pressure is the force of blood flow against the inner walls of the arteries. When that force becomes stronger than normal and can potentially harm the arteries, it's called high blood pressure or hypertension.

contain high concentrations of cholesterol. Very-low-density lipoproteins (VLDL) and larger particles called chylomicrons contain a higher proportion of triglycerides. In general, LDL, VLDL, and chylomicrons move fats from the gut and the liver to the rest of the body, while HDL moves fats from the body to the liver, where they are packaged for excretion. That's why HDL is called "good," and LDL is known as "bad." VLDL plus LDL plus HDL equals your total cholesterol, which is measured after fasting. (Chylomicrons appear only after a meal.)

When the different lipoproteins exist in normal proportions, they are not a health risk. However, when total cholesterol or LDL levels rise, or the amount of HDL drops, the body has a tendency to deposit cholesterol in the arteries. Although triglycerides do not accumulate in arteries like cholesterol does, abnormally high levels of triglycerides also are associated with an increased risk of heart attack and stroke.

### Take Action Against High Cholesterol

Although low levels of HDL increase cardiovascular risk, efforts to raise HDL have not proven beneficial. That's why physicians promote taking action against LDL

cholesterol and triglycerides, since lowering levels of these lipids have a positive impact on the heart.

Cleveland Clinic cardiologists advocate LDL levels under 100 mg/dL for many people who have not had a heart attack, and 70 mg/dL or less for those who have. These are lower than previous recommendations because clinical trials have confirmed that the lower your level of LDL, the lower your risk of having a heart attack or stroke, developing unstable angina, or needing stenting or CABG.

Accumulations of plaque start at a young age and grow over time. Since even slightly elevated cholesterol levels in adults ages 35 to 55 lay the foundation for developing heart disease, you shouldn't wait until you are older to worry about cholesterol. Lowering LDL beginning early in life is more effective in reducing risk than lowering LDL with a statin later in life. The increased benefit appears to be independent from how LDL is lowered. This means that diet and exercise are probably as effective as statins or other medications at reducing the risk of CAD when started early in life.

Next to quitting smoking, the next best thing you can do to prevent a heart attack

## Cholesterol and Triglyceride Guidelines

Cleveland Clinic cardiologists follow very aggressive guidelines for managing cholesterol levels. In this chart, we compared them with the National Cholesterol Education Program's (NCEP) guidelines. Although Cleveland Clinic guidelines recommend lower target levels of LDL, total cholesterol and triglycerides, everyone agrees that it is most important for patients to do everything they can to achieve optimal LDL levels. Both Cleveland Clinic and the NCEP advise starting a low-cholesterol, low-fat diet even if you do not have heart disease, have fewer than two heart disease risk factors, and your LDL is less than 160 mg/dL.

All cholesterol values are given in milligrams per deciliter (mg/dL)

| | | LDL [a] | Total cholesterol | HDL [b] | Triglycerides |
|---|---|---|---|---|---|
| CLEVELAND CLINIC | People without heart disease | <100 | <150-175 | Men: >40 / Women: >50 | <150 |
| | People with heart disease | <70 | <150 | Men: >40 / Women: >50 | <150 |
| NCEP | People without heart disease | <160 | <200 | >40 | <150 |
| | People with heart disease | Moderate risk: <130<br>High risk: <100<br>Very high risk: <70 | <200 | >40 | <150 |

[a] Neither Cleveland Clinic nor the NCEP consider lowering total cholesterol to these levels a therapeutic goal. This is because LDL typically makes up 60 to 70 percent of total serum cholesterol. If LDL targets are met by lifestyle modifications and/or medical therapy, it's almost certain that total cholesterol levels will fall accordingly.
[b] The NCEP has not issued guidelines for raising HDL to a specific goal, although it recognizes low HDL as an independent risk factor for coronary artery disease. NCEP guidelines simply define low and high levels, and encourage adoption of lifestyles and/or drug therapy to raise HDL as part of an overall treatment plan to manage other lipid risk factors, particularly LDL.

is to get your cholesterol down to recommended levels. Start by eating a diet low in saturated fats and trans fats. Saturated fats raise LDL. Trans fats raise LDL and total cholesterol and lower HDL. The most common sources of trans fats are hydrogenated fats, such as shortening, margarine, and partially hydrogenated cooking oils. Virtually all fried foods plus many bakery goods and snack foods are high in trans fats. When you eliminate these foods, adding nuts to your diet is one thing you can do that might lower your cholesterol.

If you have high triglyceride levels, you may want to take high-dose supplements of the omega-3 known as eicosapentaenoic acid (EPA)—especially if you have cardiovascular disease or diabetes and one additional risk factor (see "Stronger Dose of Omega-3 Significantly Reduces CV Risk").

## High Blood Pressure

High blood pressure (hypertension) greatly increases your risk of stroke, heart attack, heart failure, and kidney failure at any age. Although the incidence of hypertension increases with age, high blood pressure is not a natural part of aging. Even if you are over age 80, blood pressure-lowering treatment can reduce the risk of stroke or transient ischemic attack (TIA, or "mini-stroke") by 30 percent, death from stroke by 39 percent, death from any cause by 21 percent, death from heart attack by 23 percent, and risk of heart failure by 64 percent.

Widely fluctuating blood pressure may be as dangerous as stable high blood pressure, emphasizing the need to keep blood pressure under consistent control. Hypertension is dangerous because it forces the heart to pump harder to push blood into and through the arteries. When it pumps so hard for a long time, the heart muscle initially compensates by growing thicker, like a weightlifter's biceps. However, this adaptation only works for so long. The heart eventually becomes an increasingly ineffective pump. High blood pressure also is believed to damage the lining of the coronary arteries

and arteries throughout the entire body, providing sites where fatty plaques can form and cause atherosclerosis. Lowering blood pressure by modifying diet or taking medication gives the arteries a chance to heal and return to their normal, healthy state.

Hypertension guidelines divide patients at risk into four categories (see "Revised Categories Mean You May Now Have Hypertension"). Your overall risk also depends on the presence of other risk factors and diseases. People in the pre-hypertension range are at increased risk of developing hypertension, for which medication will be required. This can be avoided by adopting healthy habits that bring down or at least stabilize blood pressure.

Depending on your blood pressure, your doctor may first recommend changes in diet and exercise before prescribing an antihypertensive drug, since increasing activity can lower blood pressure and eliminate the need for medication. Even if your doctor prescribes a drug to lower your blood pressure, the following guidelines may be suggested:

- **Lose weight.**
- **Limit your alcohol consumption.**
- **Get regular aerobic exercise.**
- **Get enough potassium,** calcium, and magnesium in your diet by eating dairy products, bananas, sweet potatoes, green vegetables, and nuts.
- **Other foods and beverages,** including low-calorie cranberry juice and flaxseed, may have a beneficial effect on blood pressure.
- **Restrict sodium intake.**

The average American diet contains the equivalent of two to four teaspoons of table salt per day. Reducing that amount to one teaspoon normalizes blood pressure for many people with mild hypertension and may even prevent or delay the development of hypertension in healthy people. Anyone diagnosed with hypertension, all African-Americans, and everyone age 50 and older should strive to reduce sodium intake to no more than a teaspoon, or 1,500 mg, a day.

Be aware that daily use of pain-relieving medications, such as nonsteroidal anti-inflammatory drugs (NSAIDs: Advil®, Motrin®, Voltaren®, Aleve®, Naprosyn®, Celebrex®), puts you at risk for developing hypertension. Aspirin can be used as an occasional pain reliever, but should not be taken to prevent a first heart attack or stroke without first discussing it with your doctor. (It will, however, help you prevent a second heart attack, if you've had one already.)

## Diabetes Mellitus

The association between diabetes mellitus and atherosclerosis is so strong that if you have diabetes, chances are very good that if you do not control your risk factors, you will develop CAD.

Diabetes mellitus is basically a disorder of sugar metabolism. The body absorbs sugar from food and converts it into a form it can store and use for energy between meals. The blood transports absorbed sugar to your liver, muscles, and fat tissue for conversion into starch and fat. The pancreas, a gland located next to the stomach, produces a hormone called insulin when blood sugar levels increase after a meal. Insulin acts on the cells of your body to facilitate removing sugar from the blood and moving it into cells.

Type 2 diabetes is a risk factor for heart disease linked to obesity, high blood pressure, and high cholesterol. For reasons not completely understood, cells stop responding to insulin, no matter how much the pancreas makes. This is called insulin resistance. You will be diagnosed with insulin resistance if your fasting blood glucose level is between 110 and 126 mg/dL. If it's above 126 mg/dL, you have type 2 diabetes.

Drugs that keep a tight lid on blood sugar have reduced some of the complications of

## Blood Pressure—Where Do You Fit In?

Blood pressure is given as two numbers representing millimeters (mm) of mercury (Hg, the chemical symbol for this element). For example, 90/60 is read as "ninety over sixty." Because the pumping part of the cardiac cycle is known as systole (SIS-tuh-lee), the first number is referred to as the systolic (sis-TALL-ick) pressure. The filling part of the cardiac cycle is known as diastole (di-AST-uh-lee), so the second number is called the diastolic (di-uh-STALL-ick) pressure.

The risk of cardiovascular disease (CVD) doubles with every 20 mmHg increase in systolic blood pressure (BP) above 120 mmHg. Because there is strong evidence that lower blood pressure is generally better—particularly in patients with, or at high risk, for CVD—target blood pressures were lowered last year. Although blood pressure readings considered normal (optimal) did not change, more people are now considered to have hypertension (HTN).

| OLD CATEGORY | SYSTOLIC / DIASTOLIC | NEW CATEGORY | |
|---|---|---|---|
| Optimal blood pressure | Under 120/under 80 | Normal blood pressure | Under 120/80 |
| Prehypertension | 120-139/80-89 | Elevated | 120-129/ under 80 |
| Stage 1 hypertension | 140-159/90-99 | Stage 1 | 130-139/80-89 |
| Stage 2 hypertension | 160-179/100-109 | Stage 2 | 140+/90+ |
| Stage 3 hypertension | 180+/110+ | | |

*Journal of the American College of Cardiology, May 2018*

## Diabetes Mellitus

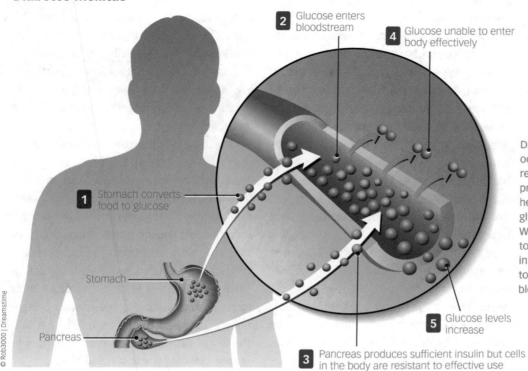

**2** Glucose enters bloodstream

**4** Glucose unable to enter body effectively

**1** Stomach converts food to glucose

Stomach

Pancreas

**5** Glucose levels increase

**3** Pancreas produces sufficient insulin but cells in the body are resistant to effective use

© Rob3000 | Dreamstime

Diabetes mellitus, or type 2 diabetes, occurs when the body no longer responds to the hormone insulin produced by the pancreas. Insulin helps "unlock" cells to take in glucose (sugar) from the blood. When the cells become resistant to insulin, more glucose remains in the bloodstream. When there is too much glucose circulating in the blood, the result is diabetes.

type 2 diabetes, but heart attack and stroke remain responsible for 65 percent of deaths in these patients. These drugs, called insulin-sensitizing agents or anti-hyperglycemic agents, enhance insulin sensitivity. By doing so they enable the cells to remove sugar from the bloodstream with less insulin. In this case, however, obtaining just the right blood sugar level is important, as very low blood sugar levels (hypoglycemia) that result in hospitalization have been identified as a risk factor for cardiac death.

Since people with type 2 diabetes are especially prone to developing CAD, they must be treated more aggressively if they also have high cholesterol or high blood pressure (see "Three Diabetes Drugs Shown to Reduce Cardiovascular Risk"). Losing weight—as little as 10 pounds—can stop or reverse insulin resistance. High blood pressure, high cholesterol levels, and high triglyceride levels often disappear along with the pounds. Conversely, most longtime type 2 diabetes patients who do not make the necessary lifestyle adjustments will eventually require insulin therapy.

## Type 1 Diabetes

Type 1 diabetes is very different from type 2. It is an autoimmune disease that generally starts in childhood, when the immune system mistakenly attacks the cells in the pancreas that make insulin. This prevents the pancreas from making enough insulin

**NEW FINDING**

### Three Diabetes Drugs Shown to Reduce Cardiovascular Risk

Type 2 diabetes greatly increases the risk of developing cardiovascular disease, which can lead to a heart attack, stroke, amputation, kidney failure or blindness, often at an early age. Medications that normalize blood sugar levels can help prevent or delay the development of atherosclerosis in the arteries. But after someone with type 2 diabetes is diagnosed with cardiovascular disease, there are only three drugs that can reduce the risk of a cardiovascular event or death. Empagliflozin (Jardiance®) was the first. It was approved by the U.S. Food & Drug Administration (FDA) in December 2016 after clinical trials showed it reduced cardiovascular mortality in patients with diabetes. It is taken as a daily pill.

In August 2017, liraglutide (Victoza®) was approved for lowering the risk of heart attack, stroke, and cardiovascular death by 13 percent. Liraglutide is injected once a day though a pre-filled pen.

In October 2018, the FDA approved canagliflozen (Invokana®) for reducing the risk of a cardiovascular event or death by 14 percent in the overall population with diabetes and by 18 percent in diabetic patients with cardiovascular disease. The oral medication also is available in fixed-dose combinations with metformin (Invokamet®) and metformin extended-release (Invokamet XR®).

or making it at all. Patients with type 1 diabetes require insulin injections under the skin.

Most studies on the impact of diabetes on the heart have made no distinction between type 1 and type 2—participants were simply lumped together as "having diabetes." But recent research examined patients with type 1 separately and found they were at very high risk for heart problems. In fact, type 1 diabetes may be as bad for the heart as type 2, or worse. Even when controlled well with insulin, type 1 diabetes was found to increase the risk of heart failure four times. Poorly controlled type 1 diabetes raised the risk 10 times. Once kidney damage occurred, the risk of heart failure increased 18 times. This suggests people with type 1 diabetes should take steps to lower all cardiovascular risk factors, in addition to keeping their blood sugar under control.

## Metabolic Syndrome

CAD is more likely to occur in patients who exhibit a specific constellation of risk factors that often appear together. The constellation constitutes metabolic syndrome, and more than 50 million Americans have it. Metabolic syndrome is defined as the presence of three or more of the conditions. The risk of heart attack and other cardiac events compounds with the addition of each risk factor, because the risk factors foster the formation of atherosclerosis. The underlying risk factors for metabolic syndrome are abdominal obesity and insulin resistance. Other contributing factors are inactivity, aging, hormone imbalance, and a genetic predisposition to insulin resistance.

Lowering cardiac risk involves treating the individual components of metabolic syndrome by losing weight and eating a diet low in saturated fat and cholesterol and high in fiber (30 grams a day recommended); increasing physical activity; quitting smoking; and taking blood pressure medication, if required. Reducing stress through activities such as meditation or exercise may help. However, studies have shown that bad habits adopted in stressful times, rather than stress itself, may be responsible for the increased risk.

## Obesity

Regardless of whether you are pear-shaped, apple-shaped, or big all over, being overweight is dangerous. Obesity is not just a risk factor for CAD. It also increases your risk of developing high blood pressure, type 2 diabetes, stroke, gallbladder disease, and cancer of the breast, prostate, and colon. Of these, high blood pressure may pose the greatest risk, accounting for more than 30 percent of excess heart attack risk and 65 percent of excess stroke risk. Obesity is now considered by many to be the second-leading preventable cause of death in this country after smoking. It's also common: More than 68 percent of U.S. adults and 31.8 percent of children ages two to 19 are overweight or obese.

A good way to figure out if you are obese is to calculate your body mass index or ask your doctor to calculate it for you. If you fall into the overweight or obese categories, you should seriously consider modifying your lifestyle by changing and restricting your diet and by taking up exercise to lose weight safely and keep it off. If you

### Some Diet Drugs Increase Heart Attack Risk; Others May Not

Research has shown that overweight patients with cardiac risk factors and/or type 2 diabetes who took the diet drug sibutramine (Meridia®) had a 16 percent increased risk of heart attack and stroke, even when they followed a diet-and-exercise program. The likely reason is that sibutramine increases blood pressure and resting pulse rate, both of which increase the risk of heart attack or stroke. The intended results might not be long-lasting enough to justify the risk: Study participants lost only about 9.5 pounds the first year, then regained weight before achieving a net weight loss of 8.8 pounds.

Lorcaserin (Belviq®), a newer drug, was approved for weight loss in addition to diet and exercise. Its possible impact on heart attack and stroke risk is still being studied.

The combination of phentermine and topiramate XL (Qsymia®) may be safer. Qsymia is approved for obese patients or overweight patients with at least one additional cardiovascular risk factor. In studies, patients using Qsymia lost an average of 6.7 to 8.9 percent of their body weight. Although study participants taking the drug experienced a significant increase in heart rate, this appeared to be offset by a drop in blood pressure.

are morbidly obese (100 pounds over your ideal weight if you're a man; 80 pounds if you're a woman), a weight-loss drug might be needed. These drugs also are useful for patients who cannot exercise due to physical limitations or for "jump starting" the weight-loss process. Be sure to discuss this option with your physician because some diet drugs actually can increase your risk of heart attack.

It is important to note, however, that even normal-weight people who carry fat in their belly have a higher death risk than obese individuals.

The primary cause of obesity is the consumption of more calories than are burned through exercise. Between 1972 and 2004, the average calorie consumption jumped by 22 percent in women and 10 percent in men. Much of this was due to larger portion sizes. The source of calories matters, too, and many of those calories came from carbohydrates (starches, refined grains, and sugars), fast foods, and sugar-sweetened beverages and snacks. Equally concerning, the American Heart Association reports that 30 percent of adults do not engage in any physical activity at all.

## Your Diet

The fact that so many people are overweight or obese should not reassure you that carrying extra weight is acceptable. The good news is that losing only 10 percent of your body weight—a "doable" goal—can help drop your heart risk from high to medium of from medium to low.

There are lots of diets to choose from. Many have a scientific basis, while others are fad diets that may do more harm than good. The American Heart Association and National Cholesterol Education Program recommend a diet in which only eight to 10 percent of calories come from saturated fats, 10 percent or less from polyunsaturated fats, and 15 percent or less from monounsaturated fats. Get advice from your doctor and other reputable sources such as the American Heart Association; the National Heart, Lung, and Blood Institute; and the U.S. Department of Agriculture. If dieting on your own doesn't work, consider joining a weight-loss program or find a registered dietitian to create a diet just for you.

Even if you are not overweight, changing your diet to make it healthier can lower your risk of CAD. Depending on your eating habits, a complete dietary overhaul may be necessary, especially if you eat Southern-style foods. Fried chicken, fried fish, fried potatoes, bacon, ham, liver, gizzards, and sweet tea increase the risk of developing cardiovascular disease.

## Mediterranean Diet

One diet known to have cardiovascular benefits is the Mediterranean diet. It is rich in fish, olive oil, fruits and vegetables, and low in animal fats that promote atherosclerosis. The Mediterranean diet contains about 30 percent fewer calories from saturated fat and 50 percent less cholesterol than the average Western diet. It is also higher in fiber and antioxidants, such as omega-3 and omega-6, which, when consumed in foods may safely slow the development of atherosclerosis in the coronary arteries and elsewhere (see "Mediterranean Diet Reduces Stroke Risk").

## DASH Diet

The DASH diet comes from a major government study called Dietary Approaches to Stop Hypertension (DASH). This study found that people who emphasized fruits, vegetables, and low-fat dairy products in their diets reduced saturated and total fat consumption and cut back on sodium significantly. Research on this diet has been so positive that some experts regard it as one of the most important non-drug measures for controlling hypertension.

The DASH eating plan was developed for people with a systolic blood pressure of 160 mmHg or less and a diastolic blood pressure of 80 to 95 mmHg, but is now considered an appropriate heart-healthy diet for any individual. You can learn more about the DASH eating plan by downloading, "Guide to Lowering Your Blood Pressure with DASH" from https://www.nhlbi.nih. gov/files/docs/public/heart/new_dash.pdf.

### Other Heart-Healthy Diets

Diets high in certain types of seafood also appear to be protective. Fatty fish contain omega-3 unsaturated fatty acids, which do not raise blood cholesterol levels. These fatty acids make the blood thinner and less sticky, reducing the risk of blood clots and inflammation that are thought to facilitate the growth of plaques. Eating as little as one meal a week of a fatty fish, such as fresh or canned tuna, salmon, mackerel, trout, or halibut, might reduce the risk of heart attack by 50 to 70 percent. Be sure to prepare your fish by baking or broiling it, since frying negates any cardiovascular benefits.

A vegetarian diet also can lower a person's risk of heart disease by one-third. In the largest study to compare cardiovascular disease rates between vegetarians and people who ate meat and fish, the vegetarians had a 32 percent lower risk of hospitalization or death from cardiovascular disease than people who consumed meat or fish.

Researchers also have found that daily doses of probiotics typically found in yogurt and other dietary supplements may lower cholesterol.

A diet that includes ample antioxidants also is thought to help protect against heart disease. Antioxidants neutralize certain highly toxic molecules called oxygen free radicals. They are produced by cells consuming oxygen while metabolizing sugars for energy. Free radicals are not all bad—they attack bacteria and help prevent infections. Yet if they are not neutralized by antioxidants, they attack healthy cells and tissues, causing extensive damage that fosters atherosclerosis. Smoking, consuming excessive quantities of alcohol, eating a high-fat diet, getting too much sun, and being exposed to polluted air all increase the generation of free radicals by our bodies.

Foods naturally high in antioxidants include yellow and orange vegetables and fruits, such as carrots, sweet potatoes, apricots, peaches, and strawberries; dark green leafy vegetables, such as broccoli and spinach; vegetable oils; citrus fruits; tomatoes, garlic, nuts, and olives. Unfortunately taking antioxidant vitamins are

---

## Bariatric Surgical Procedures

Anyone with a body mass index of 35-40 and any other serious cardiovascular risk factor who has been unable to lose a substantial amount of weight on their own may be a candidate for weight-loss surgery. The two most common forms of bariatric surgery—laparoscopic sleeve gastrectomy and laparoscopic Roux-en-Y gastric bypass—have been shown to be effective in losing weight and keeping it off, resolving weight-associated comorbidities, and lowering cardiovascular risk. Both are performed through several small incisions, rather than in open surgery.

In a sleeve gastrectomy, a large portion of the stomach is removed. This limits how many calories are consumed before feeling full.

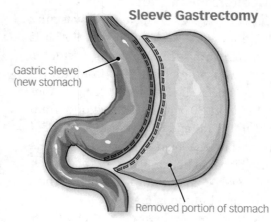

**Sleeve Gastrectomy**

Gastric Sleeve (new stomach)

Removed portion of stomach

### Roux-en-Y Gastric Bypass

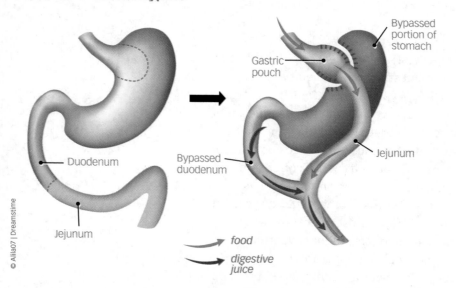

Bypassed portion of stomach

Gastric pouch

Duodenum

Bypassed duodenum

Jejunum

Jejunum

food

digestive juice

In Roux-en-Y surgery, the doctor creates a small pouch out of part of the stomach. The rest of the stomach cannot receive any food. The pouch is then connected to a part of the small intestine known as the Roux limb, forming a "Y" shape.

no substitute for these foods. They do not help lower your risk of heart disease and, in fact, may increase your risk of dying.

Certain flavonoids in purple grape juice and red wine also are powerful antioxidants. Several studies have suggested that drinking alcohol in moderation may reduce the risk of a heart attack. The benefit was first noted with red wine, but any alcoholic drink appears to afford similar protection. Just the same, possible benefits must be weighed against known risks, and most cardiologists would not encourage nondrinkers to take up alcohol, given the adverse health effects of overuse. If you don't drink alcohol, purple grape juice will help protect your heart health.

Weight loss occurs more quickly by expending calories during exercise. The heavier you are, the more difficult it may be to start an exercise program. For weight-loss purposes, lots of long, slow walks are effective.

Other effective weight-loss methods include:

- Bariatric surgery
- Structured weight-loss programs
- Regular meetings with a physician, dietitian, or weight-loss coach
- Spelling out exactly what to eat and avoid
- Receiving prepared meals or shopping lists.

## Physical Inactivity

According to the American Heart Association, the risk of developing CAD from physical inactivity is comparable to the risk associated with high blood pressure, high cholesterol levels, and cigarette smoking.

Adopting a regular program of physical activity is a good way to eliminate this risk factor. Aim for a minimum of 30 minutes of light-to-moderate exercise five days a week, or 20 minutes of vigorous exercise three days a week (see "To Live Longer, Start Walking!" on page 32).

Aerobic exercise helps prevent age-related thickening and stiffening of the arteries, as well as impairment of vascular function. Fitness also enhances the ability of individual heart muscle cells to process calcium. This improves the heart's pumping ability and reduces the risk of deadly arrhythmias. Exercise increases blood flow, which in turn increases the production of beneficial nitric oxide, reduces the number of harmful free radicals, and increases the production of antioxidants. Exercise causes certain stem cells known as endothelial progenitor cells to migrate from the bone marrow to the circulation system, where they promote the growth of small blood vessels throughout the heart and repair damaged endothelium. Exercise also slows heart failure and muscle breakdown from aging, thereby slowing the aging process.

The regularity of physical activity is more important than the intensity of the workout. You don't have to train for a marathon, and in fact, may be better off if you don't: Hard exercise does not protect against cardiac death like regular, easy exercise does. Ordinary tasks like yard work and house-cleaning, and pleasant physical pastimes such as walking and bicycling, all count as physical activity, too. They have proven to be very good for the heart, as long as they are done nearly every day.

If you are overwhelmed by the prospect of exercise, ease into it. You'll get the same benefits. As you get in shape, you'll be able to increase the duration and intensity of your workout. Start with a modest exercise program and then build up gradually to at least 30 minutes a day. If you have CAD or any risk factor for heart disease, it's a good idea to ask your doctor for advice on what kind of exercise and what intensity is ideal for you.

Finally, there's one more compelling reason to exercise: The greater your capacity to exercise, the less likely you are to have a heart attack. And if you have one, you are more likely to survive it. Fitness increases the body's ability to withstand the assault from a heart attack, lessening the amount of permanent damage to the heart.

## Physical Activity and Calories

The chart below shows the approximate calories spent per hour by a 100-, 150- and 200-pound person doing specific activities.

| ACTIVITY | 100 LB | 150 LB | 200 LB |
|---|---|---|---|
| Bicycling, 6 mph | 160 | 240 | 312 |
| Bicycling, 12 mph | 270 | 410 | 534 |
| Jogging/ Running, 7 mph | 610 | 920 | 1,230 |
| Jumping rope | 500 | 750 | 1,000 |
| Running/ Jogging 5.5 mph | 440 | 660 | 962 |
| Running/ Jogging, 10 mph | 850 | 1,280 | 1,664 |
| Swimming, 25 yds/ min | 185 | 275 | 358 |
| Swimming, 50 yds/ min | 325 | 500 | 650 |
| Tennis, singles | 265 | 400 | 535 |
| Walking, 2 mph | 160 | 240 | 312 |
| Walking, 3 mph | 210 | 320 | 416 |
| Walking, 4.5 mph | 295 | 440 | 572 |

Source: Adapted from ACSM's Guidelines for Exercise Testing and Prescription, Ninth Edition, and Ainsworth BE, Haskell WL, Herrmann SD, Meckes N, Bassett Jr DR, Tudor-Locke C, Greer JL, Vezina J, Whitt-Glover MC, Leon

## To Live Longer, Start Walking!

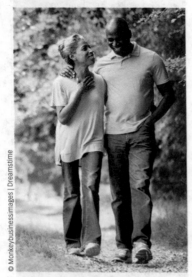

Walking at an average pace is considered a moderate-intensity activity. Walking for only two hours a week can lower your risk of death from all causes, found researchers involved in a cancer prevention study. Responses to 143,000 questionnaires revealed that people who walked "some," but "less than the recommended amount," were 26 percent less likely to die prematurely than those who reported being "inactive." Those who met or exceeded the minimum recommendations of 150 minutes a week of walking or other moderate-intensity exercise had a risk that was 20 percent lower than the rate for those who walked "some."

*American Journal of Preventive Medicine*, online Oct. 19, 2017

## Emerging Risk Factors

While one or more of the traditional risk factors just described apply to about 80 to 90 percent of all people who develop CAD, some people with no established risk factors still get the disease. The following conditions are known to be risk factors in some people. However, further studies are needed before widespread screenings can be justified.

### Low Levels of "Good" Cholesterol

Low levels of "good" HDL cholesterol are an independent risk factor for CAD, meaning that low levels increase the chance of developing CAD, even in the absence of any other risk factor. Evidence comes from studies such as the landmark Framingham Study, which showed that the risk of heart attack was higher in people with lower HDL levels. In fact, very low levels of "good" HDL may actually negate the benefits of a low LDL.

What perplexes physicians is that raising HDL with medications, such as niacin or fibrates, doesn't lessen cardiac risk. Two large clinical trials found no benefit in raising HDL when LDL was optimally treated.

What we do know is that the quality of HDL is more important than the quantity. Inflammation and oxidation can hinder its ability to remove cholesterol from artery walls and return it to the liver. When high levels of high-sensitivity C-reactive protein (hsCRP)—a marker of inflammation—are present in the blood, the risk of heart attack is high, even in patients with high levels of HDL.

### High Levels of Coronary Artery Calcium

The buildup of calcium in the coronary arteries can help predict the risk for developing serious CAD and cardiovascular events in women who are otherwise thought to be at low risk. A coronary artery calcium score (CACS) can be obtained with computed tomography. In the Multi-Ethnic Study of Atherosclerosis (MESA), the risk of a serious cardiovascular event was directly correlated with CACS; women with the highest scores were at six times the risk of those with no detectable coronary artery calcium.

It is important to note that even though there have been concerns in the medical community as to whether calcium supplements contribute to the buildup of calcium in the arteries, an expert panel concluded that it is safe for individuals to take calcium supplements for bone health without increasing the risk for cardiovascular disease.

People who live in the center of urban areas may be twice as likely to have coronary artery calcification (CAC) than people who live in less polluted urban and rural areas. Although air pollution is suspected in the development of CAC, the mechanisms by which air pollution may contribute to CAC are not well understood.

A genetic variant for lipoprotein(a), or Lp(a), a cholesterol-rich particle that circulates in the blood, also may increase the risk of heart attack and stroke as well as playing a role in calcium buildup in the heart's aortic valve (aortic stenosis), which can result in heart failure, stroke, and sudden cardiac death. A 10-fold elevation in Lp(a) due to a genetic variation can raise the risk of aortic valve stenosis by 60 percent. More severe elevations can double or even triple the risk.

### Psychosocial Factors

It is becoming clear that depression, isolation, and anger appear to be serious factors in the development of a heart attack. It also appears that depression makes you more likely to develop atherosclerosis, have a heart attack, or die from heart disease. In 2014, after an extensive review of the literature, a 12-person panel of experts recommended to the American Heart Association that depression be added to the list of risk factors associated with heart disease (see "Antidepressants May Save Lives from Post-Heart Attack Depression").

Anxiety appears to be equally risky. In fact, anxious men have four times the risk of sudden death from heart attack. Moreover, new research has found that caregivers for family members with cardiovascular disease may unintentionally raise their risk for heart disease by neglecting their own health.

Researchers have not been able to prove that these emotions actually cause plaque to form in the arteries. They suspect that depression, isolation, and anger cause chemical changes in the body that make platelets clump together and form blood clots.

Research conducted on people suffering from post-traumatic stress disorder (PTSD) identified the amygdala as the area of the brain responsible for the reaction and connects it with heart attack and stroke. The amygdala is the area that controls emotions.

People with a supportive network of family and friends are at less risk for heart attack and fare better after a heart attack or surgery for heart disease than do loners.

## Pollution

Long-term exposure to pollution may increase the risk of death for heart attack survivors, a European study found. By linking the records of 154,204 heart attack survivors between 2004 to 2007 with air pollution data from 2004 to 2010, researchers were able to assess the impact that pollution had on death rates. They found deaths increased by 20 percent in patients exposed to higher levels of tiny air pollutants that measured 2.5 micrometers in diameter, which is about 30 times smaller than a human hair. Conversely, the death rate among heart-attack survivors exposed to lower levels of air pollutants declined by 12 percent.

## Sleep

Getting too little or too much sleep can lead to heart problems, according to findings from the National Health and Nutrition Examination Survey (NHANES). Adults who get less than six hours of sleep a night are at a significantly greater risk of stroke, heart attack, and congestive heart failure.

What's more, those who sleep more than eight hours a night have a higher prevalence of heart problems, such as chest pain and CAD.

Obstructive sleep apnea (OSA) can lead to serious heart problems. OSA is characterized by abnormal pauses in breathing during sleep. These pauses can last from 10 seconds to minutes, and may occur five to 30 times or more an hour. In one study of women with OSA, researchers found that 31 percent had abnormal electrocardiograms (see page 36).

Although insufficient sleep has been linked to cardiovascular disease, researchers do not know why longer sleep duration may be linked to heart problems. The National Sleep Foundation recommends that adults should aim for at least seven hours of sleep every night.

## Certain Blood Markers

If you smoke or have high levels of traditional modifiable risk factors for heart disease, you will need to make lifestyle changes and/or take medications to lower your risk of heart attack. But these measures only reduce heart attacks by about 50 percent.

Researchers have looked for additional ways to improve risk prediction. Many substances in the blood have been identified as possibilities. Only a small number of these biomarkers have been proven useful enough to be widely adopted. Today, abnormally high levels of six substances in the blood are used to provide additional help in identifying people who remain at risk, so they can be treated more aggressively:

### High-sensitivity C-Reactive Protein

C-reactive protein (CRP) is a marker or sign of inflammation in the body. When measured by a high-sensitivity (hs) laboratory test, high levels of CRP are associated with a higher risk of CAD and heart attack, even in patients with normal cholesterol levels. The test is useful for identifying patients with elevated risk that was not identified with traditional tests, who remain at risk

NEW FINDING

**Antidepressants May Save Lives from Post-Heart Attack Depression**

Depression after a heart attack can have serious, even deadly, consequences. However, treatment with the selective serotonin reuptake inhibitor (SSRI) escitalopram (Lexapro®) may significantly reduce the risk of a major cardiac event. In one study, patients who had recently suffered a heart attack were randomized to the antidepressant or placebo for 24 weeks. All-cause deaths, deaths from heart disease, heart attacks, and revascularizations with angioplasty and stenting were tracked for a median of eight years. At this point, 40.9 percent of the patients on escitalopram and 53.6 percent on placebo had suffered one of these adverse events. The SSRI beat placebo in all individual outcomes, but only reduction in heart attack (8.7 percent vs. 15.2 percent) was statistically significant.

*Journal of the American Medical Association, July 24/31, 2018*

## New Drug Fights Heart Disease in a New Way

The role of trimethylamine N-oxide (TMAO) in heart attack and stroke was discovered by Cleveland Clinic researchers in 2015. The same researchers have now created a new class of drugs that prevent gut bacteria from making TMAO without harming the microbes, which are generally beneficial. These drugs, known as mechanism-based inhibitors, trick the bacterial cells into thinking they are nutrients and absorbing them. Once they are inside the cell, these drugs block the production of TMAO. When tested in mice, a single dose of the new drug reversed platelet reactivity and excessive clot formation for three days, after which it simply remained in the gut and continued to target its microbe. This new class of drugs has the potential to reduce deaths from cardio-vascular disease and is being tested in human clinical trials.

*Nature Medicine*, Sept. 2018

Ejection fraction is the percentage of blood in the ventricles pumped out with each beat. A normal ejection fraction is 55 to 65 percent. The lower the percentage, the more advanced the heart failure.

despite statin therapy, or who might need more aggressive therapy to reduce the risk of a heart attack.

### Lipoprotein(a)

Abnormally high blood levels of a lipoprotein related to LDL called lipoprotein(a), or Lp(a), appear to confer an increased risk of CAD and heart attack in men under age 55 and in all women, especially those over age 55. High levels of Lp(a) are genetically determined, so high Lp(a) levels indicate higher risk in patients with a strong family history of CAD. Because Lp(a) is attached to LDL cholesterol, aggressive LDL lowering is necessary to lower the risk of heart attack.

### Homocysteine

An amino acid called homocysteine contributes to the development of heart attack and stroke in people with no recognized risk factors. Every 10 percent increase in homocysteine levels increases risk of CAD by 10 percent. Homocysteine is necessary for normal cell function. Under certain circumstances, excess homocysteine leaks out of cells and into the blood, where it may damage the endothelial cells lining the arteries and provide a site for atherosclerosis to develop. Currently, homocysteine is used primarily to identify patients with chronic kidney disease who are at increased risk for a cardiac event and require aggressive blood pressure and cholesterol reduction.

### Myeloperoxidase (MPO)

MPO is a marker of inflammation in the blood vessels. High MPO levels signify an increased risk of heart attack, even when HDL, LDL, and hsCRP levels are normal. MPO is a protein secreted by white blood cells to kill bacteria. Its presence inflames arteries, changes LDL into a form that causes plaques to develop, and prevents HDL from doing its beneficial job. It also releases a type of "bleach" that kills cells in the artery lining, causing plaque to become unstable and reducing the ability of nitric oxide to relax blood vessels. High levels of MPO in people with heart disease or chest pain indicate very high risk of heart attack. High MPO levels are treated with aggressive antiplatelet and LDL-lowering therapy.

### Trimethylamine N-oxide (TMAO)

TMAO is a compound produced when bacteria in the gut digest certain nutrients found in meat, egg yolks, and high-fat dairy. TMAO makes blood platelets prone to clotting. High levels of TMAO are known to be a strong predictor of increased risk for heart attack or stroke caused by a blood clot. Fortunately, a new class of drugs with exciting potential to counteract TMAO is being tested in clinical trials (see "New Drug Fights Heart Disease in a New Way").

### N-terminal pro-brain natriuretic peptide (NT-proBNP)

BNP is a hormone that causes blood pressure to rise and the body to retain sodium and water. High levels of NT-proBNP indicate worsening left ventricular ejection fraction, making the test valuable for diagnosing heart failure in asymptomatic patients. High NT-proBNP levels require blood pressure to be tightly controlled.

## Committing Yourself

If you're interested in lowering your risk of CAD, or you have been diagnosed with CAD or found to be at high risk of having a heart attack, it may be hard to rid yourself of unhealthy habits that you've had for years and adopt new, heart-healthy ones. But it's in your best interest to do so. Studies have shown convincingly and repeatedly that the more heart-healthy habits you adopt, and the longer you maintain them, the more you will reduce your risk, no matter how old you are when you start.

If you're at high risk, your doctor will probably start you on medications and recommend that you make lifestyle modifications to lower your risk. Commit yourself to heart-healthy habits, and you'll find that the drugs you take will be more effective in lowering your risk.

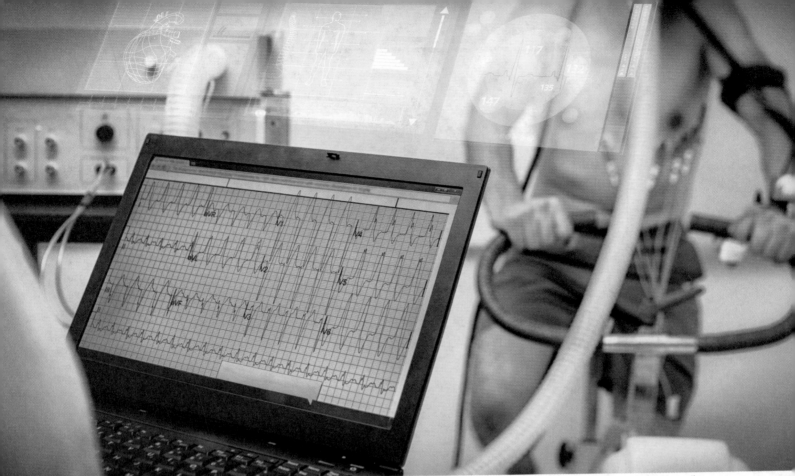

## 4 Detecting and Diagnosing CAD

If you have risk factors or symptoms suggestive of a heart attack, your doctor will want to run some tests. A variety of diagnostic tests are used to help determine the presence and extent of CAD, as well as the risk of having a heart attack. The tests your doctor chooses will depend in part on your symptoms and the urgency of your situation. An emergency department visit for acute pain requires a different approach than mentioning to your doctor that you have occasional chest discomfort when you exert yourself. Either way, your doctor will want to know if the discomfort is caused by CAD, how many and which coronary arteries are affected, and how severely blood flow is restricted. Some physicians may use newly developed methods to determine if your plaques are stable or prone to rupture. The results will determine the most appropriate treatment.

There are two categories of diagnostic tests for CAD: non-invasive and invasive.

Non-invasive tests quickly assess the heart's condition from outside the body, and are usually done first when the situation is not an emergency.

Invasive tests are more complicated and expensive, and require special probes and equipment. Invasive procedures are not practical or cost-effective for screening for CAD, so they are generally reserved for people with worsening symptoms consistent with narrowed coronary arteries or abnormal results from non-invasive testing. A physician may order an invasive test when non-invasive tests suggest CAD has progressed to the point where stenting or bypass surgery may be needed.

### Non-Invasive Diagnostic Tests

The most commonly used non-invasive tests to diagnose CAD are electrocardiography, stress tests, nuclear perfusion tests, and echocardiography.

An exercise stress test (above) is one of several screenings that help doctors diagnose heart disease.

## The ECG Recording

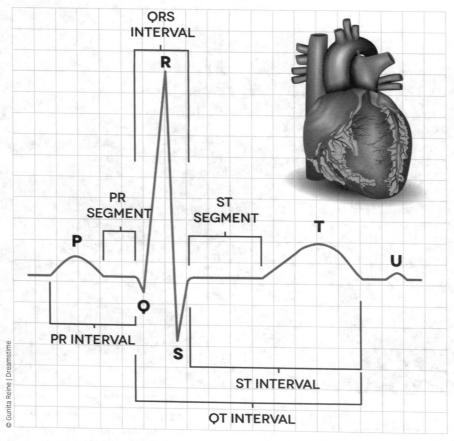

© Gunta Reine | Dreamstime

The heart's own pacemaker cells contract in response to impulses that originate in the sinoatrial (SA), or sinus, node. The first heart muscles to contract are the atria, which propel the blood into the ventricles. The impulse reaches the atrioventricular (AV) node, where it is slightly delayed to give time for this flow to occur. The AV node then amplifies the impulse and sends it on its way through the ventricles, stimulating them to contract and propel the blood out of the heart. The heart muscle then relaxes and gets ready for the next heartbeat.

The ECG records the heartbeat as a series of electrical oscillations designated P, Q, R, S, and T waves. The P wave is the impulse that stimulates atrial contraction. The Q, R, and S waves represent the impulse that stimulates ventricular contraction. The T wave represents the relaxation of the ventricle. A normal heart rate is 60 to 100 beats per minute. The duration of each cycle is about three-quarters of a second, and it becomes even shorter as the heart beats faster during exercise.

### Electrocardiography

Electrocardiography provides a snapshot of the electrical impulses that make up your heartbeat. The recording of your heart's electrical activity is called an electrocardiogram (ECG, or EKG from the German elektrokardiogramm). Changes from the normal, expected pattern can reveal evidence of old heart attacks, a heart rhythm disturbance, an enlarged heart, or other problem. However, a normal ECG does not necessarily mean you do not have CAD.

### Stress Tests

Because chest discomfort from CAD is usually triggered by exertion, your doctor may want to take an ECG while your heart is being stressed. The most common type of stress test involves walking on a treadmill or riding a stationary bicycle. Evidence of CAD may appear on the ECG as you approach your limit of exercise capacity. By comparing your ECG before, during, and after exercise, your doctor will have a much better idea of the extent and severity of your CAD.

If you have stable angina, your ability to perform a stress test will be limited. Nevertheless, you may be asked to undergo additional stress tests periodically, since any changes in your performance could provide clues to whether your CAD is getting worse, or whether medical therapy and lifestyle changes are improving your condition.

### Nuclear Perfusion Tests

A stress test conducted after a radioactive isotope has been injected is called a nuclear perfusion ("blood flow") test or scan. The radioisotope—usually thallium or technetium—is carried by the blood and accumulates in portions of the heart that have adequate blood flow. When CAD is blocking a coronary artery, the thallium or technetium can't get through. This test helps reveal whether all parts of the heart muscle are receiving adequate blood flow.

The radiation emitted by these radioisotopes are gamma rays, so a camera that sees only gamma rays is used to image the heart at rest and after exercise. The technique is called Single-Photon Emission Computed Tomography (SPECT); "single-photon" because the radioisotope emits only one wavelength of gamma radiation. A camera collects these rays, and a computer constructs an image from the emitted radiation. Tomography is a method of reconstructing cross-sectional images (slices) of the heart, to evaluate blood flow to the myocardium (heart muscle). Normal flow throughout the myocardium at rest and with exercise argues against the presence of severe CAD. Normal flow at rest that decreases after exercise suggests a severe coronary artery narrowing. Decreased flow both at rest and during exertion tends to indicate scarring from a past heart attack.

An exercise nuclear perfusion scan can help identify patients with severe CAD, a group at high risk for heart attack. Those who show poor blood flow are then treated appropriately in hopes of preventing a heart attack. When a person cannot exercise, adenosine (Adenoscan®) or dipyridamole (Persantine®®),or r Regadenosoin (Lexiscan®)e is given through a vein to "dilate," or open up, the coronary arteries. Vessels that are heavily diseased cannot dilate as much as healthy ones, selectively decreasing the delivery of the radioactive tracer to the heart muscle. Of note, a typical nuclear stress test provides a radiation dose equivalent to 900 chest X-rays.

## Echocardiography

An echocardiogram ("echo") is a collection of moving pictures of the heart taken with very high-frequency sound waves (ultrasound). Echocardiograms reveal the shape, size, position, and motion of cardiac structures, including the thickness of ventricle walls, the condition of heart valves, or the presence of abnormal openings between the chambers.

Echocardiography can provide two-dimensional (2-D) or three-dimensional (3-D) images. The more commonly used 2-D echo technology provides moving pictures of slices of the heart. These pictures are usually taken from the front of the heart through the chest wall in a technique known as transthoracic echocardiography (TTE). Under certain circumstances, pictures also may be taken from the back of the heart via the esophagus in a procedure

**Echocardiography**

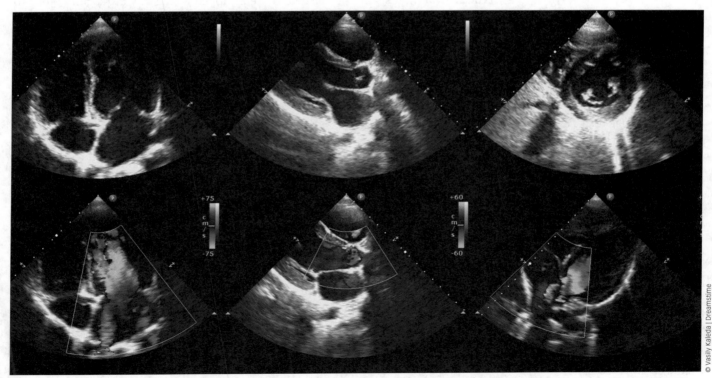

© Vasily Kaleda | Dreamstime

Echocardiography is a type of ultrasound that uses high-pitched sound waves to create moving images of the heart. It's especially helpful in detecting problems with the valves or chambers of the heart.

called transesophageal echocardiography (TEE). During heart surgery, TEE is often used to assess the heart's pumping function or to confirm whether a valve repair or replacement has been successful.

A sophisticated emerging technology known as 3-D echocardiography provides more information by reconstructing the heart on a computer screen. The 3-D image can be rotated to view the heart from different angles.

Stress echocardiography is often used as an indirect test for CAD. Patients either exercise on a treadmill or receive a drug called dobutamine that makes the heart beat faster and harder. If the walls of the heart do not contract as well during stress as they do at rest, blockages may be limiting blood flow to the hard-working heart muscle.

## Invasive Diagnostic Tests

Invasive diagnostic tests help confirm the presence of CAD, identify which coronary artery or arteries are obstructed, and determine whether stenting or bypass surgery is needed. Invasive tests are performed in a cardiac catheterization laboratory (cath lab). The gold-standard test for diagnosing severe CAD is selective coronary angiography, a method of taking x-ray movies of the beating heart and its arteries that was developed at Cleveland Clinic.

### Angiography

To perform angiography, a thin, flexible tube called a catheter is inserted into a blood vessel in the groin, elbow or wrist and advanced to the mouth of the coronary arteries. This procedure is called cardiac catheterization. A liquid contrast material ("dye") that blocks x-rays is injected through the catheter directly into the coronary arteries, enabling the internal contours of the coronaries to be clearly seen. These images, called angiograms, are viewed in real time and digitally recorded. Coronary arteries that are narrowed or completely blocked by plaque can be immediately identified on the angiograms.

Coronary angiography is performed primarily on:

▶ **Patients with stable or unstable angina and severe or worsening symptoms,** and patients who have had a heart attack. Often, the condition of these patients has not improved with medical therapy, so they are being considered for stenting or coronary artery bypass surgery.

▶ **Patients with symptoms that suggest CAD,** but whose diagnosis has not been confirmed by non-invasive diagnostic procedures.

▶ **Patients who have undergone non-invasive testing with results that suggest the presence of severe lack of blood flow to the heart muscle (ischemia),** even in the absence of angina. This condition, called silent myocardial ischemia, may be as dangerous as the CAD that causes angina.

### Intravascular Ultrasound (IVUS)

Intravascular ultrasound (IVUS) uses a catheter tipped with a tiny ultrasound probe to take pictures inside the coronary arteries using high-frequency sound waves. IVUS provides a direct look at the size and composition of plaques, and is particularly valuable for monitoring plaques as they change over time or when overlapping arteries cause a fuzzy image on an angiogram.

A tiny ultrasound transducer on the tip of the IVUS probe bounces sound waves off the walls of the coronary arteries and sends signals back to a computer, where they are immediately translated to images and displayed on a monitor. These images show the artery walls, the central channel (lumen) through which blood flows, and the presence or absence of plaque. Different types of plaque reflect sound waves in different ways, enabling the cardiologist to tell whether the plaque is mostly hard or soft.

It is particularly valuable when coronary angiography is unable to determine if a lesion is blocking the artery 70 percent or more—the point at which treatment with angioplasty or bypass surgery may be required.

With this information, they are better able to choose the most appropriate treatment and size of stent for holding the artery open. After a stent has been inserted, IVUS may be used to ensure it is fully expanded. IVUS also is used in clinical trials to monitor the effects of cholesterol-lowering and anti-inflammatory medications on plaque.

## Recent Advances in Non-Invasive and Invasive Diagnostic Testing

Several innovative methods of examining the heart are now being assessed to see if they can provide information in a less-invasive and, hopefully, less-expensive way.

### Computed Tomography Angiography (CTA)

Angiography conducted with computed tomography (CTA) already has proven invaluable in studies of arteries in the brain, lungs, kidneys, arms, and legs. Some leading cardiologists feel that CTA has the potential to become an accurate, non-invasive method of imaging the coronary arteries.

CTA is performed with high-powered scanners with dual-source technology, which enables images of the heart and coronary arteries to be obtained in seconds. The speed of these scanners significantly reduces image blur generated by the fast motion of the beating heart.

It can identify older, harder plaques by their calcium content, producing a calcium score. The higher the score, the more severe the CAD and the greater the risk of heart attack. The newest CT scanners also reveal plaques without calcium, which may be more vulnerable to rupture.

CTA is sometimes used in place of cardiac catheterization. But just when CTA is a better choice is unclear. In a large study

## Computed Tomography Angiography

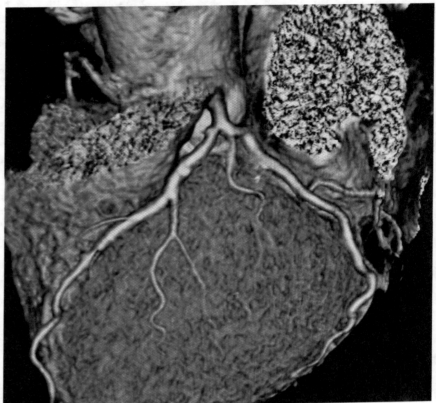

Computed tomography (CT) angiography provides more anatomical detail of the heart than other imaging techniques. It is particularly useful for assessing the size of the aorta. In younger patients without significant coronary calcification, it can be used to assess coronary artery disease.

of more than 10,000 patients with symptoms suggestive of CAD, CTA was no better than traditional stress testing for diagnosing CAD. However, CTA can be effective in evaluating the coronary arteries of patients with suspected dilated cardiomyopathy, a form of heart failure that is not caused by narrowing of the coronary arteries. In these patients, CTA is correct 99 percent of the time in ruling out CAD.

In 2010, several medical organizations issued joint guidelines for the use of cardiac CT. They deemed the use of cardiac CT appropriate for diagnosis and risk assessment in patients at low or intermediate risk, to gauge probability of CAD or to evaluate the structure and function of the heart. Other appropriate uses include CT without contrast for calcium scoring in low- and intermediate-risk patients with a

## Positron Emission Tomography (PET) Scanning

A type of nuclear imaging called positron emission tomography (PET) is one way to tell the difference between stunned (in shock) heart muscle and nonfunctional scar tissue.

When blood flow to heart tissue is completely stopped, healthy tissue dies and is replaced by scar tissue. However, temporary blockage of blood flow—such as what happens during a heart attack—can cause the heart muscle to go into shock. Although it appears dead, the muscle is only stunned. The concept of stunned heart muscle is easy to understand with this simple analogy: Sitting too long in one position can impinge on a nerve. When you stand up, your leg does not move normally for several minutes. The heart responds the same way when it has been deprived of oxygen. Sometimes, when a trickle of blood is able to keep stunned heart muscle alive for a prolonged period of time, the muscle is said to be hibernating. This is of great interest to cardiologists, because hibernating heart tissue usually recovers when its blood supply is restored.

In PET scanning, a short-acting radioactive tracer called rubidium is injected into the bloodstream, and the patient is scanned with a nuclear camera. Normal heart muscle absorbs the radioactive agent, but scar tissue and hibernating muscle do not. However, hibernating muscle will take up radioactively tagged sugar molecules in the area where rubidium was not absorbed. If the scan shows the heart muscle is receiving normal blood flow, chances are good the patient's discomfort stems from a source other than the heart.

## Optical Coherence Tomography (OCT)

Optical coherence tomography (OCT) produces highly accurate images of the artery wall using the reflection from light rays. Various tissue components reflect light differently, enabling all tissue layers to be clearly differentiated from each other. OCT

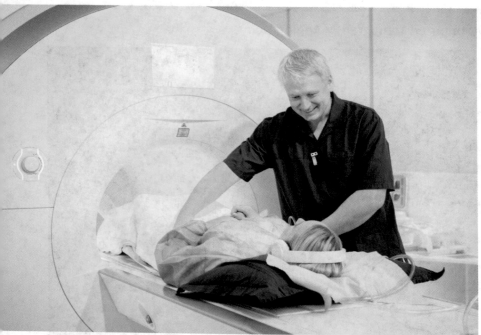

© Leaf | Dreamstime

A cardiac CT scan is a painless screening that can reveal if there is blockage in the coronary arteries.

family history of premature CAD, for pre-electrophysiology testing, and before repeat CABG or valve surgery.

Inappropriate applications of cardiac CT include its use in high-risk patients when repeated testing is required (due to cumulative radiation exposure), for screening asymptomatic patients, and for preoperative risk assessment in patients with no history of heart conditions undergoing non-cardiac surgery.

## Magnetic Resonance Imaging (MRI)

MRI is a safe, painless, non-invasive technology that uses magnetic fields and radio waves to see inside the human body. Physicians have finally discovered a way to use MRI to identify the composition of plaque, as well as to assess the area of tissue damage following a heart attack. Cleveland Clinic cardiologists consider cardiac MRI a very useful technology and one especially suited to identifying tissue in the heart that is alive after a heart attack. It also is excellent for defining the structure of the heart, such as the size, location, and connections of the heart's chambers and great vessels (aorta, vena cava, and their branches).

can be used to determine the thickness of the fibrous cap, as well as contact between a stent and its vessel wall. However, blood flow to the artery must be temporarily stopped to conduct the test. Despite the outstanding image quality provided by OCT, it is not widely used in the United States at this time.

## Fractional Flow Reserve

This is a type of stress test done in the cath lab during a cardiac catheterization. The test uses a wire inside the heart to measure the pressures on both sides of a blockage to determine its functional significance. This test has been extensively studied and is used to determine who would benefit from a stent or CABG.

## Blood Tests

C-reactive protein (CRP) is a marker of inflammation, meaning that it indicates the presence of inflammation somewhere in the body. Inflammation is associated with the development of atherosclerosis and the rupture of vulnerable plaques—an occurrence that precipitates a heart attack. An inexpensive test to measure CRP levels in the blood known as high-sensitivity CRP (hsCRP) can be helpful in refining individual estimates of the risk of developing CAD and the risk of having a second heart attack. The higher the CRP level, the higher the risk. CRP levels can be decreased through weight loss, exercise, smoking cessation, dietary modification, aspirin, and statins.

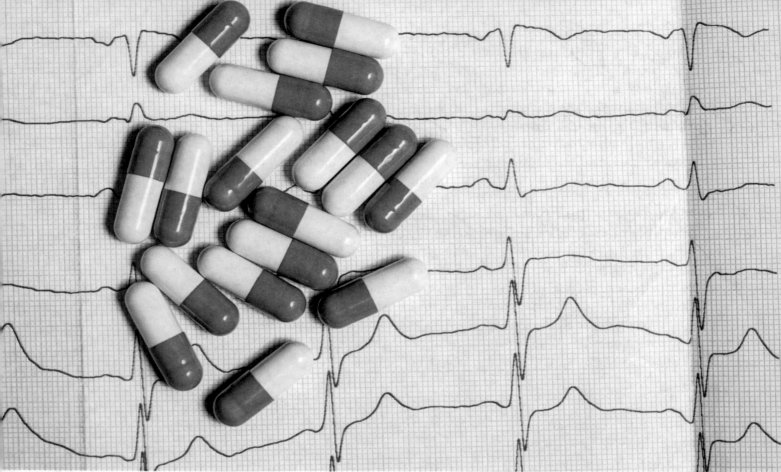

© Germanberta27 | Dreamstime

For people with CAD, medications to help control cholesterol, blood pressure, and blood glucose often are part of an overall treatment program.

Studies have shown that people who do not fill their prescriptions after suffering a heart attack are far more likely to die within a year than those who fill their prescriptions and take the medications as prescribed.

## 5 Medical Therapies

If you have stable or unstable angina or have had a heart attack, chances are you'll need to do more than modify your lifestyle to reduce your risk. Your cardiologist will need to determine if medication is needed, or if an interventional procedure is necessary to improve blood flow to your heart muscle. Cardiologists take many factors into account when trying to determine the best treatment for a patient.

If you develop chronic stable angina, intensive medical therapy may be tried first. If you develop unstable angina, you're more likely to undergo an interventional procedure.

Your doctor also may prescribe medications if you have abnormal cholesterol and/or triglyceride levels, high blood pressure, or diabetes. Be aware that taking medications to lower your risk does not mean you can go back to your bad habits: If you give up eating a low-fat diet because

you are taking a cholesterol drug, you'll gain weight and increase your cardiovascular risk. Remember, the drugs you take will be more effective if you maintain a heart-healthy lifestyle.

### Drugs to Normalize Blood Lipid Levels

Several drugs are available to help lower total cholesterol, LDL, and triglycerides and to raise HDL. Statins are the most widely used lipid-lowering drugs. PCSK9 inhibitors are much newer and more powerful. Other drugs include cholesterol absorption inhibitors, niacin, fibrates, and bile acid sequestrants.

### Statins

Statins usually lower total cholesterol by 16 to 45 percent and LDL by 20 to 60 percent in several weeks. Their effect can be boosted through the addition of soluble fiber (such as Metamucil® or psyllium, which can be purchased in health food and vitamin stores).

All statins are effective in men and women alike, regardless of whether they have suffered heart attacks (see "Statin Benefits Outweigh Risks for Most People"). Some statins lower cholesterol further than others, and some have additional beneficial properties. Cleveland Clinic researchers found that maximum doses of rosuvastatin and atorvastatin are similarly effective in reversing the buildup of cholesterol plaques in the coronary artery walls after 24 months of treatment. Your doctor will decide which statin and dose is most appropriate for you. Statins also can reduce triglyceride levels by 25 to 30 percent, but have a negligible impact on raising HDL levels.

Overwhelmingly positive results from large, well-designed clinical trials show that statins reduce fatal and non-fatal heart attacks, strokes, and the need for revascularization in people with CAD and have a wide range of other beneficial effects. Studies have shown that every 40 mg/dL reduction in LDL achieved with statins is associated with a 19 percent reduction in cardiac death and a 12 percent reduction in all-cause mortality and fewer strokes, heart attacks, and revascularization procedures. How much a person benefits from statin therapy depends on individual risk of having an event and how low a level of LDL is achieved. The lower the LDL level,

the greater the benefit, particularly when blood pressure levels are normal (less than or equal to 120 mmHg), too (see "The Lower the LDL, the Better").

Statins also benefit healthy men and women with elevated cholesterol by preventing first heart attacks. They probably do this by stabilizing the core of soft atherosclerotic plaques, making them less likely to rupture.

## Risks and Benefits

Overall, statins are safe. Their multiple beneficial effects are enduring. Side effects are generally minimal and include muscle pain or weakness (myalgia). When side effects occur, most people simply stop taking the drug. However, the risk of heart attack increases exponentially when statin therapy is discontinued.

Statins are so valuable in reducing the risk of heart attack and stroke, that European experts issued a consensus statement advising physicians how to treat these patients. Their advice was first to stop the offensive drug for two to four weeks, then try a different statin. A Cleveland Clinic study found 70 percent of patients who could not tolerate two statins, could tolerate a third that was tried. A different study found that 92 percent of patients were still taking the second statin one year later.

An alternative is to try a lower dose of a powerful statin or take the statin only two or three times a week. Some patients find that muscle pain can be controlled by

NEW FINDING

### The Lower the LDL, the Better

The benefits of low LDL cholesterol have been firmly verified in clinical trials of statins and other lipid-lowering drugs. In these trials, deaths from coronary artery disease, heart attack, stroke and revascularization dropped as LDL levels declined. For this reason, an LDL level of 70 mg/dL or lower is advised for anyone with cardiovascular disease. Yet just how low LDL levels can go and remain safe and effective has been unknown until recently. When researchers analyzed data from large clinical trials where these drugs were used alone and in combination to achieve LDL levels as low as 21 mg/dL, they found cardiovascular events continued to drop without incurring any serious adverse events.

*JAMA Cardiology*, online Aug. 1, 2018

NEW FINDING

### Statin Benefits Outweigh Risks for Most People

The potential benefits of statins far outweigh the risks, a review of 17 years of statin studies concluded. Researchers examined the incidence of several serious side effects attributed to statins and weighed them against known benefits. Statins were associated with one case of new-onset diabetes per 1,000 patients per year, but prevented three to five new cardiovascular events per year in the same population. No evidence was found that statins have adverse effects on cognitive function or cause any form of dementia or Parkinson's disease. Risk of harm to the kidneys was minor. The researchers did see a small increased risk of hemorrhagic stroke in patients with a history of ischemic stroke who take high doses of atorvastatin, but statins significantly reduced the risk of ischemic stroke.

*European Heart Journal*, online April 27, 2018

taking high doses of coenzyme Q10, which is available over the counter at pharmacies.

Patients who experience muscle pain when taking statins should visit their doctor to make sure the pain is related to statin treatment and to take a blood test that rules out rhabdomyolysis, a rare but extremely serious disease that causes muscle tissue to break down.

### What You Need to Know About Statins

Patients taking statins used to require routine periodic monitoring of liver enzymes. Today, liver enzyme tests are only performed before starting statin therapy and if indicated thereafter.

Statin labels carry a warning about the potential for generally non-serious and reversible cognitive side effects, such as memory loss and confusion, as well as reports of increased blood sugar and glycosylated hemoglobin (HbA1c) levels.

There are some situations in which lovastatin should not be used, or should be used in limited doses, when taken with certain medicines that can increase the risk for muscle injury. Also, you should limit your alcohol intake and tell your doctors if you start an antibiotic or anti-fungal medication, since it may adversely affect your liver if taken with a statin. If you have any questions or concerns about statins, ask your physician.

### PCSK9 Inhibitors

Whereas statins (HMG-CoA reductase inhibitors) reduce cholesterol by blocking the enzyme in your liver (HMG-CoA reductase) responsible for making cholesterol, PCSK9 inhibitors suppress a particular enzyme involved in determining how much cholesterol the liver eliminates from the body.

The FDA has approved two PCSK9 inhibitors: alirocumab (Praluent®) and evolocumab (Repatha®). Unlike statins, which are generally taken daily, these PCSK9 inhibitors are given as injections once every two to four weeks.

PCSK9 inhibitors are so powerful that when they are combined with statins, they can lower LDL cholesterol to rock-bottom levels. In the FOURIER study, the addition of evolocumab to statin therapy had a 15 percent lower risk of heart attack, stroke, coronary death, need for revascularization, and unstable angina requiring hospitalization than patients taking statins alone. This makes the PCSK9 inhibitor highly valuable for people with LDL levels that are two, three, or four times normal due to genetic conditions, and gives patients with genetically high cholesterol a chance to prevent heart disease. PCSK9 inhibitors can also be used alone in patients who cannot achieve adequately low LDL levels on statins alone and in patients who cannot tolerate statins due to side effects.

Despite their excellent LDL-lowering ability, PCSK9 inhibitors have the disadvantage of being expensive. Some patients have difficulty getting their PCSK9 prescription approved.

### Cholesterol Absorption Inhibitors

Ezetimibe (Zetia®), a cholesterol absorption inhibitor, works by reducing the amount of cholesterol absorbed through the digestive tract. Ezetimibe was developed for use in addition to statins and is not as effective as a statin when used alone. In studies, patients who were unable to reach their LDL goal on statins alone were able to reduce their LDL level an additional 25 percent by adding ezetimibe. Studies showed it can reduce total cholesterol by about 13 percent, LDL by 18 percent, and triglycerides by 8 percent, and will slightly increase HDL.

The IMPROVE-IT trial compared the combination of simvastatin and ezetimibe (Vytorin®) to simvastatin alone in 18,144 patients admitted to the hospital with heart attack. The addition of ezetimibe resulted in a small but significant decrease in cardiovascular events.

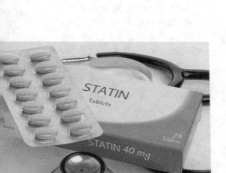

Statins are cholesterol-lowering drugs that are among the most-prescribed medications in the world.

## Niacin

Niacin, or nicotinic acid, is a component of the vitamin B complex (vitamin B3), which has been used since the 1950s to modify cholesterol levels. When taken in large doses, niacin may lower LDL by as much as 25 percent—an effect similar to that of the lower-potency statins. Cardiologists used to give niacin to raise HDL. However, a large-scale, NIH-funded clinical trial (AIM-HIGH) was halted early in May 2011 when the addition of niacin to a statin did not reduce the risk of heart attack or stroke over treatment with a statin alone. Another recent large trial (HPS2-THRIVE) yielded similarly discouraging results. As such, niacin is no longer used to raise HDL, but it can be utilized in combination with a statin to lower LDL to its desired goal.

Niacin can be used safely without statins. The downside is that niacin's common side effects—skin flushing and itching—can be bothersome enough that up to one-third of patients discontinue taking it. These uncomfortable side effects can be largely avoided by using extended-release formulations, such as Niaspan®, or by taking low-dose aspirin 30 to 60 minutes before niacin. Also, avoiding alcoholic beverages or hot beverages such as coffee or tea two to three hours before taking niacin will help reduce flushing. It is best to take niacin with food and at bedtime.

Although over-the-counter niacin formulations may be attractive to many patients seeking a "natural" alternative to cholesterol treatment, remember that such brands are considered dietary supplements and are not subject to the same federal regulations as prescription drugs like Niaspan®. Preparations listing "nicotinic acid" in the contents have the active ingredient you want. If the label says "no-flush" or "flush-free" niacin, or if the contents list "inositol hexaniacinate" as an ingredient, don't buy it. Although they sound like a great idea, these products have no detectable biological effect in humans and will not change your cholesterol levels.

### How to Minimize or Prevent Statin-Related Side Effects

Statins are generally well tolerated. However, a small percentage of patients experience side effects, usually in the form of muscle pain or muscle weakness. People with underlying muscle or gallbladder disease are at increased risk for these problems, as are statin users who drink alcohol.

Cleveland Clinic cardiologist Leslie Cho, MD, consulting editor for this publication, is a world expert on statin intolerance. She says there are three things you should try that may prevent or minimize statin-induced muscle issues, so you can continue taking advantage of these beneficial drugs.

#### 1. Check for Interactions

Make sure that no other medication you take is causing the problem. Many common antibiotics and antifungal medications, the hypertension drugs diltiazem and verapamil, and the antiarrhythmia medications amiodarone and digoxin can cause statins to linger in the body, which can trigger symptoms.

Additionally, alcohol consumption can inhibit statin elimination from the body.

#### 2. Try a Different Statin

Ask your doctor if you should change statins. Pravastatin (Pravacol®) and rosuvastatin (Crestor®) are less likely to affect the muscles than the other four statins. Dr. Cho advises her patients to stop the offensive statin for two to four weeks, then start a different statin. In a Cleveland Clinic study, 70 percent of patients could tolerate the second statin. In a different study, 92 percent of patients were still taking the second statin a year later.

#### 3. Try a Different Dosing Regimen

A little statin is better than no statin at all, so start with the lowest dose of pravastatin or rosuvastatin once a week. Gradually move to twice a week, then to three times a week. Take time to assess how well you tolerate the medication and learn how it affects your cholesterol. If you can tolerate statin therapy one, two, or three times a week, but it's not enough to help you reach your desired LDL goal, consider adding a non-statin lipid-lowering agent such as ezetimibe (Zetia®).

#### Switch to a Different Class of Drugs

If these tactics don't work, try a different class of drugs. Bile acid sequestrants with or without ezetimibe may be beneficial. A PCSK9 inhibitor—evolocumab (Repatha®) or alirocumab (Praluent®)—may be even better. These new drugs are more expensive than other cholesterol-lowering medications, but they do not tend to trigger symptoms in patients who have suffered from statin intolerance.

#### Don't Give Up

Don't try these tactics without consulting your doctor first. However, they increase the likelihood you'll be able to take a statin without experiencing side effects that are so unpleasant you need to stop taking the medication.

"Stopping statin therapy is not a good idea, since it greatly increases the chance of having a heart attack. Don't give up until you've tried all options," says Dr. Cho.

### Fibrates

Fenofibrate (Tricor®, Antara®) and gemfibrozil (Lopid®) are more effective at lowering triglycerides and raising HDL than they are at lowering LDL. Fibrates are generally used only in selected patients, particularly those with mixed hyperlipidemias (elevations in both triglycerides and LDL).

Fibrates have been shown to lower the risk of cardiovascular events by 10 percent and coronary events by 13 percent. The studies included both primary and secondary prevention patients with and without cardiovascular disease. The trials also found that fibrate therapy reduced coronary events and was well tolerated. However, the combination of statins and fibrates can increase the likelihood of muscle pain three- to five-fold.

## Bile Acid Sequestrants

Bile acids are made by the liver from cholesterol and stored in the gallbladder for release following a meal. They are necessary for the absorption of lipids from food. It is important to understand that our bodies cannot break down cholesterol—we can only get rid of it by eliminating it in the stool. Most bile acids are absorbed and reused, but bile acid sequestrants prevent this from happening. Micronized colestipol (Colestid®), colesevelam (Welchol®), and cholestyramine (Questran®) are polymers that bind to bile acids in the small intestine and prevent their reabsorption. Thus, the liver makes new bile acids, which consume more of the body's cholesterol stores. Bile acid sequestrants reduce total cholesterol, LDL, and triglycerides, and increase HDL. They are not as potent as statins, niacin, or ezetimibe, so they are normally used only in patients who are intolerant of more effective drugs or those who require a third or fourth agent to reach their LDL goal.

## Drugs That Lower Blood Pressure

High blood pressure is a risk factor for the development of CAD. Consistent use of blood pressure medications to bring blood pressure down to normal levels can lower the risk of heart attack and stroke. For this reason, major medical societies recommend maintaining a systolic blood pressure of 140 mmHg or less.

A major clinical trial known as SPRINT found that lowering blood pressure to less than 120 mmHg in patients at high risk of coronary artery disease may lower the combined risk of heart attack, stroke, heart failure, and cardiovascular death an additional 25 percent. When these endpoints were examined individually, the benefits were even more striking.

While achieving a systolic blood pressure as low as 120 mmHg may have benefits, the corresponding drop in diastolic blood pressure has risks. Doctors are now being warned that patients' diastolic blood pressure should not be allowed to drop below 70 mmHg, and never below 60 mmHg.

Many antihypertension medications are available. If one drug doesn't do the job, your doctor will try another. A combination of two or more different types is common when blood pressure resists control. A few months of trial and error may be needed to find the right drug or combination that works best for you and has the fewest side effects.

## Diuretics

Diuretics make the kidneys excrete more salt, and because water tends to follow the salt, more water is also excreted. Diuretics enhance the effectiveness of other antihypertension drugs. Many diuretics are available in generic form.

## Beta Blockers

This class of drugs prevents the hormone adrenaline (also called epinephrine) and related compounds from raising heart rate and cardiac output. They do this by blocking adrenaline from interacting with one of its cellular receptors, called a beta-adrenergic receptor. As a result, blood pressure drops.

Whether a beta blocker is right and appropriate for you depends on your medical history. Since beta blockers can sometimes cause fatigue, weight gain, depression, and erectile dysfunction, they are not first-line drugs for all patients with hypertension.

## Calcium-Channel Blockers

For muscle cells to contract, dissolved calcium must quickly enter cells through protein channels in the cell membrane. Restricting or blocking the entry of calcium hinders the muscles' ability to contract. When the muscle is surrounding an artery, the artery cannot constrict as much, which keeps blood pressure from increasing. Calcium-channel blockers (CCBs) "plug" the calcium channel.

As a warning, if you take a CCB, the antibiotics clarithromycin, erythromycin, or telithromycin may increase the risk your blood pressure will drop to dangerously low levels.

## ACE Inhibitors and ARBs

Angiotensin-converting enzyme (ACE) inhibitors reduce the production of a compound in the blood called angiotensin II, which constricts arteries and raises blood pressure. Angiotensin II receptor blockers (ARBs) prevent angiotensin II from binding to its receptors on blood vessels. They are as effective as ACE inhibitors at lowering blood pressure and may have the unique quality of preventing dementia.

An analysis of multiple clinical trials published in 2012 showed that ACE inhibitors were associated with a 10 percent reduction in all-cause mortality over four years in patients with hypertension. Patients taking other blood pressure-lowering drugs did not have this advantage.

For patients with peripheral artery disease and intermittent claudication (pain in the calf that occurs while walking and disappears with rest), 24 weeks of treatment with the ACE inhibitor ramipril (Altace®) has been associated with improvement in pain-free and maximum walking times and the physical health aspect of quality of life that reduces cardiovascular risk. In one small pilot study, ramipril was associated with a 77 percent increase in average pain-free walking time and a 123 percent increase in maximum walking time.

People who take ACE inhibitors or ARBs should have their kidney function closely monitored. Even rather small rises in creatinine levels are associated with increased risk of end-stage kidney disease, heart attack, heart failure, or death, and require the drug to be stopped.

## Combinations

To help patients with high blood pressure manage their drugs, several combinations of different antihypertension drugs, as well as hypertension drugs with other heart medications, are available in a single tablet. These combinations can be highly effective in preventing heart attack and stroke, and they simplify pill taking.

## Drugs to Reduce Risk from Diabetes

People with diabetes are at greatly increased risk for cardiovascular disease. The good news is that certain medications to control diabetes may lower your risk of heart failure, and may even protect you from cardiac death.

If you are taking drugs to control glucose levels, you also should be taking statins and aspirin, even if your lipid profile is normal or close to normal, and treating high blood pressure aggressively.

## Medical Management of Chronic Stable Angina and Unstable Angina

If you have any risk factor for CAD, atherosclerosis is likely to progress. It is very important to take steps to stop or slow this progression before you develop symptoms of CAD, such as chest discomfort, likely triggered by exertion or anxiety and relieved by rest. This is important, because most heart attacks don't come with a warning: Only 20 percent of heart attacks are preceded by symptoms of angina. About 50 percent of men and 64 percent of women who die suddenly from CAD have no symptoms of the disease.

---

### Commonly Used Calcium-Channel Blockers

Commonly used calcium-channel blockers (CCBs) that act on the small arteries of the body include:

- amlodipine (Norvasc®)
- felodipine (Plendil®)
- nifedipine (Adalat CC®, Procardia XL®)

Other CCBs act predominantly on the heart to slow its rate and force of contraction. These include:

- diltiazem (Cardizem®, Tiazac®, Dilacor XR®)
- verapamil (Calan®, Covera®, Isoptin®, Verelan®)

---

### ACE Inhibitors and ARBs

**Commonly prescribed ACE inhibitors include:**

- captopril (Capoten®)
- quinapril (Accupril®)
- ramipril (Altace®)
- benazepril (Lotensin®)
- fosinopril (Monopril®)
- enalapril (Vasotec®)
- lisinopril (Prinivil®, Zestril®)

**Common ARBs include:**

- losartan (Cozaar®)
- valsartan (Diovan®)
- irbesartan (Avapro®)
- candesartan (Atacand®)
- telmisartan (Micardis®)

If you experience symptoms, your doctor probably will order a complete battery of tests. The results will help determine your treatment. If your symptoms are not too severe, relatively infrequent, relieved by rest, and predictable based on the level of exertion, then you probably will be diagnosed with chronic stable angina.

## Chronic Stable Angina

Chronic stable angina is chest pain that occurs with exertion and disappears with rest. If you are diagnosed with chronic stable angina, your doctor will first try to determine your level of risk, which will dictate the treatment you need. More than likely, you will not need invasive treatment, as angioplasty and stenting have not been shown to be better than optimal medical therapy at improving survival.

Your doctor may make adjustments in your current medications or add medications. More than likely you will be prescribed nitrates, a beta blocker or a calcium-channel blocker, aspirin, and a statin. Or your doctor may prescribe ranolazine (Ranexa®), which is approved for patients with chronic angina who do not respond to other antiangina medications.

It is important to bear in mind that chronic stable angina is not a death sentence. About 6.4 million men and women in the U.S. have it, with about 400,000 new cases diagnosed every year. Many lead long, useful lives after the diagnosis, even after a heart attack. Although the angina may not disappear completely, many patients learn how to prevent it from interfering with their activities.

### Nitrates

These important and useful drugs prevent and relieve angina by rapidly relaxing and dilating the coronary arteries, as well as veins throughout the body. Resistance to blood flow diminishes, so blood and oxygen delivery to the heart muscle increases, while the workload of the heart decreases. These effects reduce angina.

Several nitrates are available, including nitroglycerin, isosorbide dinitrate (Isordil®), and isosorbide mononitrate (Imdur®). They are available in oral, extended-release capsules and in transdermal patches for absorption through the skin. Nitroglycerin is the most rapidly acting nitrate. A pill dissolved under the tongue provides rapid relief of angina. A metered spray (Nitrolingual Pumpspray®) also is available for spraying nitroglycerin under the tongue. Nitroglycerin degrades rapidly on exposure to air, so it must be kept in a cool, dark place and replaced when it reaches its expiration date.

Relief should begin to occur within one or two minutes, but the effect only lasts about an hour. Nitroglycerin also can be taken in anticipation of angina—usually five or 10 minutes before any physical activity or emotional stress that might spark an episode.

### Beta Blockers

Beta blockers are used to treat hypertension, but they also are effective in preventing angina during exercise, reducing the incidence of cardiac events, and improving survival rates after a heart attack in patients with stable angina.

Certain medical conditions can make use of a beta blocker risky, however, so patients with stable angina should not take beta blockers if they also have:

- A very slow heart rate (severe bradycardia), including a condition that blocks the transmission of electrical signals from the atria to the ventricles called high-degree atrioventricular block
- Atria that beat abnormally or irregularly (sick sinus syndrome)
- Severe, decompensated left ventricular heart failure
- Severe asthma or chronic obstructive pulmonary disease (emphysema or chronic bronchitis)

### Calcium-Channel Blockers

Calcium-channel blockers, another family of antihypertension medications, are used in patients who cannot take beta blockers, or for whom beta blockers are ineffective in managing their angina.

Nitrates and beta blockers or calcium-channel blockers are often more effective when used together. The most effective combination appears to be a slow-release or long-acting calcium-channel blocker of the dihydropyridine type (for example, amlodipine [Norvasc®]) plus a beta blocker. On the other hand, a beta blocker in combination with one of the nondihydropyridine calcium-channel blockers, such as diltiazem (Cardizem®) or verapamil (Covera-HS®), can cause bradycardia and low blood pressure, which in turn can make you very tired. However, diltiazem and verapamil may be effective in treating stable angina when beta blockers cannot be used or tolerated.

## Aspirin

Cheap, readily available and widely tolerated, aspirin outperforms newer heart medications in some patients. An antiplatelet medication, aspirin prevents platelets from sticking together and forming blood clots. Since blood clots can block blood flow in coronary arteries during unstable angina and heart attack, aspirin is useful in preventing angina from evolving into something more serious and life threatening. Aspirin has unequivocally been shown to reduce deaths from heart attack in multiple large studies.

As a word of caution: Although aspirin is available over the counter, it is a powerful medication, and taking too much of it may increase the risk of major bleeding.

If you have stable angina, your doctor will likely prescribe low-dose daily aspirin unless you have stomach distress, are prone to heartburn, or have had an ulcer. If so, a medication to block the release of stomach acid may be needed for aspirin to be tolerated. For people with aspirin allergies, clopidogrel (Plavix®), ticagrelor (Brilinta®) or prasugrel (Effient®) are alternatives. Anyone at higher risk for heart attack may benefit from taking one of these drugs in addition to aspirin.

In some patients, aspirin fails to prevent platelets from sticking together. The term "aspirin resistance" has been coined to explain this phenomenon. Other patients are resistant to clopidogrel. While this may occasionally occur, new thinking is that some patients simply need higher doses of these medications to prevent blood clots. In too many cases, blood clots occur because patients stop taking these medications without their doctor's permission.

## Unstable Angina

When angina occurs suddenly and is not relieved by rest, it is called unstable angina (UA). UA is an emergency, since it can deteriorate into a heart attack in a flash.

Identifying a heart attack is not always easy. Symptoms of heart attack can be vague, and the symptoms may be caused by other, less serious conditions. When a patient arrives in the emergency department with a suspected heart attack, tests are done to distinguish UA from a milder heart attack known as a non ST-segment elevation myocardial infarction (NSTEMI, caused by partial blockage of a coronary artery) and a more severe heart attack caused by a total blockage in the coronary artery (STEMI). Until the difference is known, the patient is said to have ACS.

The principal difference between UA and NSTEMI is the severity of the blockage. ECGs obtained from patients with UA and NSTEMI are almost identical, except that abnormalities indicating the heart is not receiving enough oxygen tend to be temporary in unstable angina and persistent in NSTEMI.

When an artery is blocked, injured heart muscle cells spill certain proteins called troponins into the blood. Troponins are normally kept inside the cells, so it's a sign that the cells are beginning to die. Troponin

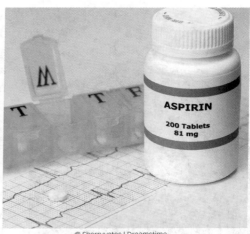

© Sherryyates | Dreamstime

Aspirin is an antiplatelet medication that can be used to help keep angina from progressing to a heart attack. Low-dose or "baby" aspirin may also help prevent heart attacks in people already diagnosed with heart disease.

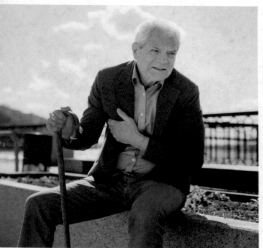
© Zinkevych | Dreamstime

Angina is temporary chest pain brought on by a narrowing of the coronary arteries.

levels can be measured by a simple blood test that provides a quick, accurate answer. If the proteins appear, a diagnosis of NSTEMI is made. If not, it's UA. Since elevated troponin levels indicate damage to the heart and increase the risk of death, cardiologists take a more aggressive approach to treatment when these markers appear.

## When Angina Worsens

If you have stable angina and experience any worsening in the frequency, duration, or intensity of angina, or if your angina occurs with less exertion than before, it's possible that your CAD has advanced. Call your doctor immediately. If you have angina at rest and you can't get relief from rest or nitroglycerin, call 911.

Medical treatment of UA is the same as for stable angina, except the dose of beta blocker or calcium-channel blocker may be increased, and nitroglycerin may be given intravenously. These treatments will be closely monitored to prevent your heart rate from slowing down too much or your blood pressure from dropping too low.

In addition, you will probably be given an infusion of a blood thinner to prevent a life-threatening blood clot in your coronary arteries. You'll also be given aspirin and possibly other platelet inhibitors. With medical therapy, up to 80 percent of patients improve within two days of hospital admission. However, immediate angioplasty can cut the risk of heart attack in half.

Several clinical trials have been conducted to determine whether patients with UA should be taken to the cath lab soon after hospital admission, or whether doctors should wait and see if medical therapy is effective. The "as soon as feasible" approach has been called the "early invasive" approach, while the "take the drugs and wait and see" approach has been referred to as the "conservative" approach. In the early invasive approach, the patient is given medical therapy for symptoms of UA and scheduled for a cardiac catheterization one to three days later. The choice of treatment—continued medical therapy, stenting, or bypass surgery—depends on what the cardiologist finds.

## Aggressive Treatment

Cleveland Clinic cardiologists are convinced that immediate treatment reduces deaths and complications, as well as length of hospital stay. An analysis of major trials comparing the aggressive and conservative approaches found that aggressive treatment with an invasive therapy substantially reduced subsequent heart attacks, angina, and rehospitalizations. Cardiologists are now focusing on improving procedures and pinpointing the optimal timing of an invasive procedure.

To avoid future episodes of UA or heart attack, your doctor may recommend an interventional or surgical procedure to restore blood flow through or around your blocked coronary arteries.

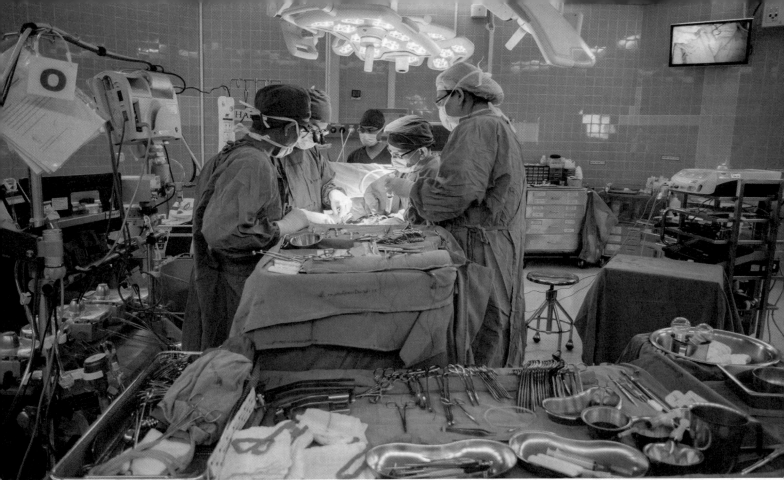

© Rufous | Dreamstime

# 6 Interventional and Surgical Treatments

Interventional cardiology procedures have greatly enhanced recovery, survival, and quality of life. Cardiac catheterization is now a routine procedure for patients with chronic angina, UA, and heart attack. When a narrowing or complete blockage is found, cardiac catheterization may be combined with a therapeutic procedure called stenting to immediately improve or restore blood flow without the trauma and delay of major surgery. Stenting, a type of percutaneous coronary intervention (PCI), is performed in the cardiac catheterization laboratory by interventional cardiologists. The procedure does not require anesthesia, although sedation may be used to relieve anxiety. An overnight stay in the hospital after the procedure is generally required.

In some patients, the extent or location of the blockages makes stenting impossible or dangerous to perform. Such patients become candidates for coronary artery bypass grafting (CABG, or bypass surgery). CABG is performed in an operating room by cardiac surgeons. The procedure requires general anesthesia. When standard open-heart surgery is performed, patients must stay up to a week in the hospital, with recovery taking up to four to six weeks. The use of minimally invasive techniques shortens the hospital stay and lessens postoperative pain.

Increasingly, hospitals are opening hybrid operating rooms (ORs), which are essentially operating rooms with the equipment needed to do a cardiac catheterization. This type of OR allows an interventional cardiologist and cardiac surgeon to work together on a patient with multi-vessel disease. In a combined procedure, the surgeon performs one or two bypasses on the most important vessels, and the cardiologist puts stents in the remaining blockages.

Procedures to treat CAD include traditional open-heart surgery as well as a growing number of less-invasive approaches using catheters or robotic surgeons.

**CORONARY ARTERY DISEASE | 51**

## Angioplasty and Stenting

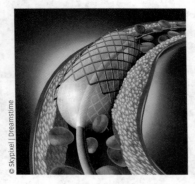

Sometimes a blocked artery can be treated with angioplasty. In this procedure, a catheter with a tiny, uninflated balloon at the tip is inserted into a blood vessel in the arm or leg and guided to the site of the blockage. The balloon is inflated and the plaque is pushed against the walls of the artery, widening the space for blood to flow. The catheter and balloon are then withdrawn. In some cases, a wire mesh tube called a stent is left behind to help keep the artery open.

PCI and CABG are some of the most frequently performed procedures in the United States. Both lifesaving procedures enable the vast majority of patients to return to, if not improve, their former lifestyle.

## Angioplasty and Stenting

Angioplasty involves positioning a catheter with an inflatable balloon at its tip inside the plaque. When the balloon is inflated, it pushes the plaque against the wall of the artery to make the inside diameter (lumen) bigger. Next, the balloon is deflated and retrieved, leaving nothing manmade in the body.

Ways of removing the plaque using cutting tools, drill bits, and lasers have been developed. In certain cases, rotational atherectomy can be valuable in re-establishing blood flow and making room for a stent. It is now complemented by newer technologies, such as the Crosser Catheter System and orbital atherectomy, which break up stubborn calcium deposits.

The most persistent problem of angioplasty is the rapid rate that plaque re-obstructs blood flow—sometimes in only a few weeks. The solution to this problem is to implant a stent inside the vessel. The tube-shaped metal mesh scaffold was designed to remain in the artery after the balloon-tipped catheter is withdrawn, physically preventing the plaque from springing back. Yet stents can become blocked by the ingrowth of new cells and scar tissue, which restricts blood flow—a process called in-stent restenosis.

To prevent unwanted cell growth, many stents are coated with chemotherapy drugs that are slowly released (eluted) into the wall of the artery. These are called drug-eluting stents (DES). Both DES and bare-metal stents (BMS) are widely used today in different patient populations.

Unfortunately, neither type of stent is perfect. For patients with simple lesions, DES may be a viable option, and the risk of in-stent thrombosis may not be much more than with BMS. Yet it can still occur.

A new type of stent called a bioresorbable vascular scaffold (BVS) can prevent in-stent restenosis altogether. Doctors are excited about these gelatin stents that dissolve over time, leaving a healthy artery behind. However, they are not suitable for all types of coronary artery blockage and have a very limited role at this time.

Because patients with DES need to stay on antiplatelet therapy for up to a year after implantation, any elective dental work or surgical procedure—hip replacement, for example—should be done before stenting. Stopping the antiplatelet drugs during the surgery will increase the risk of heart attack.

### What to Expect

You will be scheduled for an elective cardiac catheterization and possible PCI if your symptoms of CAD are worsening, your stress test indicates impaired blood flow to the heart muscle, and your cardiologist wants to get a close look at your coronary arteries.

Emergency cardiac catheterization followed by PCI will be performed when you arrive at the hospital in an ambulance with unstable angina or symptoms of a heart attack.

You will be taken to the catheterization laboratory and prepared for a cardiac catheterization. The angiogram will be used to determine the extent and severity of your blockage or blockages. If your cardiologist finds a few fairly well-defined blockages, and these sites can be reached by the catheter, the cardiologist may continue with the PCI procedure. If you have more extensive disease, you may be better suited for CABG.

PCI will feel like a continuation of the cardiac catheterization procedure and usually takes only one or two hours. When it is over, you will be moved into a telemetry unit and be monitored for complications, such as bleeding from the puncture site. You probably will be able to go home a day or two after the procedure—longer if you suffered a heart attack.

## Possible Complications

### Acute Closure

Acute closure (also called abrupt closure) is a rare complication that can happen soon after PCI—usually within minutes or hours, but sometimes within days. Acute closure is the obstruction of blood flow at the treatment site by a new blood clot, contraction of the coronary artery (elastic recoil, dissection, or rebound), or both. Whatever the cause, acute closure deprives the heart muscle of oxygen and nutrients, causing a heart attack. If this happens, the catheterization is usually repeated to examine the stent for acute clot formation (thrombosis).

Today, because most PCI patients automatically receive a stent, and because multiple oral and IV medications are given to prevent clot formation, acute closure is highly unusual.

### Restenosis

Adverse events that occur several months after stenting are usually due to narrowing of the inside of the vessel by scar tissue that has grown into the stent, a process called "in-stent restenosis." For unclear reasons, narrowing also can occur at another location in the artery. Patients who develop severe restenosis can undergo angioplasty and have a DES inserted inside an existing stent, or undergo CABG.

Although BMS significantly reduced the incidence of acute closure and restenosis, investigators several years ago believed that the presence of a foreign object—a metal tube—stimulated the cells of the coronary artery wall to overgrow into the stent. This prompted efforts to find a coating that the stent would gradually elute (release) over time to prevent restenosis. Several were tried. Gold actually increased the rate of restenosis, while heparin (an anticoagulant) had little effect. Two drugs, however, have proven to be effective: sirolimus (Rapamycin® or Rapimmune®), an immunosuppressive agent used to prevent organ rejection in patients after kidney transplantation, and paclitaxel (Taxol®),

a drug used in patients with certain cancers. When released from a stent, these drugs inhibit the proliferation and migration of cells in the coronary artery wall that cause restenosis.

Researchers are taking several different tacks in an effort to prevent restenosis. New DES are coated with one or two compounds related to sirolimus, including everolimus (Afinitor®) and zotarolimus. Other stents are made of different metals.

### Thrombosis

The benefits of DES are clear: almost complete elimination of acute closure and a reduction in the one-year rate of restenosis to less than 10 percent. The success of DES was initially tempered by the finding of increased "late in-stent thrombosis," the dangerous, potentially fatal condition of blood clot formation inside the stent a year or more after it is implanted. However, subsequent trial data showed that late in-stent thrombosis is exceedingly rare. Taking antiplatelet medications can help prevent a blood clot from occurring. The current recommendation is to take aspirin plus either clopidogrel (Plavix®), ticagrelor (Brilinta®), or prasugrel (Effient®)—a regimen known as dual antiplatelet therapy (DAPT)—for up to 12 months. Treatment can usually be interrupted at six months if noncardiac surgery is required.

After clopidogrel, ticagrelor, or prasugrel is stopped, aspirin is continued for life. Patients with bare-metal stents must take the drugs for at least 30 days, but a period of several months is preferred. Studies have found that patients who stop taking antiplatelet medications earlier than recommended have a significantly increased risk of suffering a heart attack or death. However, the drugs do increase the risk of bruising and bleeding, and can exacerbate conditions such as ulcers. Doctors must take into consideration other medications the patient is taking.

Many patients with CAD take the blood thinner warfarin (Coumadin®). However,

### What Is a Stent?

Stents are metal support tubes made of stainless steel; alloys of other inert metals, such as nickel, titanium, tungsten, cobalt, chromium, molybdenum, tantalum; nonmetallic synthetic polymers (plastics); or other materials, including papyrus. They are collapsed and placed onto the tip of a balloon catheter for threading into a coronary artery. When the balloon is inflated, the stent expands into its final shape. Stents come in several lengths and can be expanded to a certain diameter.

An expanded stent looks like a tiny tube of flexible chicken wire or chain-link fence. When deployed during angioplasty, a stent forms a supporting scaffold that prevents the coronary artery from collapsing. Some stents are coated with a drug to stop tissue from growing inside the stent; other stents dissolve and disappear over time.

**How stent deployment works:**

- A collapsed stent on a balloon catheter is threaded to the area of the plaque.
- The balloon is inflated, expanding the stent and pressing it against the plaque, causing a slight bulge in the artery.
- The balloon catheter is removed and the opened stent remains in place.

## What Is a GPIIb/IIIa Inhibitor?

GP stands for "glycoprotein," which is a protein with sugar molecules attached. IIb ("two-B") and IIIa ("three-A") are two different glycoproteins exposed on the surface of platelets that form part of the "glue" that makes platelets stick together. The other part of the glue is fibrinogen, which forms a bridge between two platelets. One end of a fibrinogen molecule sticks to GPIIb/IIIa on one platelet and the other end sticks to GPIIb/IIIa on another platelet. Imagine thousands of platelets sticking to each other this way. The clump can get big enough to plug holes in arteries or block blood flow in coronary arteries. GPIIb/IIIa inhibitors prevent fibrinogen from sticking to GPIIb/IIIa and, therefore, platelets from sticking to each another.

Supervised exercise is a key component of cardiac rehabilitation. Heart patients learn how to exercise safely at a level that will help strengthen the heart muscle and improve circulation throughout the body.

combining warfarin with dual antiplatelet therapy (DAPT) after stenting can increase the risk of unwanted bleeding. The problem is greater when taking prasugrel or ticagrelor, instead of clopidogrel. Therefore, clopidogrel should be combined with aspirin as DAPT in patients who must continue taking warfarin.

## Drugs Used Before, During, and After PCI

Before undergoing PCI, patients are given a drug regimen of anticoagulants and antiplatelet agents ("blood thinners") to minimize blood clots. The drugs may include aspirin, clopidogrel, ticagrelor, prasugrel, unfractionated heparin, the direct thrombin inhibitor bivalirudin (Angiomax®), or one of three available GPIIb/IIIa inhibitors: abciximab (ReoPro®), eptifibatide (Integrilin®) or tirofiban (Aggrastat®). These drugs work in complementary ways. Anticoagulants prevent the protein called fibrinogen from converting into strong fibers that clot blood. Antiplatelet agents prevent platelets—small cells that help start formation of a blood clot—from becoming activated and sticking together.

Daily aspirin will usually be prescribed for a few days before the procedure. And unless CABG is required in the next few days, it will be continued indefinitely, since stopping aspirin carries a high risk of heart attack. If bleeding or an allergic reaction occurs in response to taking aspirin, your physician will substitute a different antiplatelet agent.

Clopidogrel may be started at home about three days before checking into the hospital. Clopidogrel is particularly effective in patients receiving a stent, but a single large dose ("loading dose") is also recommended within six hours prior to any PCI procedure.

Once you are in the cath lab, you may be given unfractionated heparin, a direct thrombin inhibitor, or a GPIIb/IIIa inhibitor. GP IIb/IIIa inhibitors are usually reserved for high-risk PCIs. Bivalirudin may be used in place of heparin or a GPIIb/IIIa inhibitor.

After stenting, a daily baby aspirin (81 mg) and an antiplatelet agent are recommended.

## Opening Blockages with Other Methods

Many patients undergo PCI after an acute episode of unstable angina or a heart attack, since these situations strongly suggest the presence of a blood clot in a coronary artery. Removing existing blood clots before angioplasty may improve the chances of an event-free recovery.

When the clot is particularly large, using AngioJet® is an option. This device shoots a fine stream of saline into the clot to break it apart and then sucks the particles and saline back into the catheter for removal from the body.

Another method involves using aspiration catheters, which suck clots from the arteries.

Some blockages are caused by slow buildup of cement-like plaque. A technique for treating these patients is rotational atherectomy, a different form of PCI that employs a diamond-tipped drill to break through the hard plaque. In certain cases, rotational atherectomy can be valuable for re-establishing coronary blood flow and making room for a stent. It is now complemented by newer technologies, such as orbital atherectomy, which represent other methods of breaking up stubborn calcium deposits.

## Closure Devices

"Percutaneous" means "puncture," and PCI procedures are performed with a catheter that enters an artery through a puncture. If the PCI was performed through the leg, after the procedure the cardiologist will sometimes place a stitch or a collagen plug in the femoral artery. This action may decrease the period of bed rest required after the procedure, but it does not decrease the risk of bleeding. These devices cannot be used in all cases, and sometimes the traditional technique of putting pressure on the puncture site is still the most effective way to stop bleeding.

If the catheterization was performed through the wrist, no closure device is required. An inflatable wristband holds the puncture site closed and is slowly deflated until bleeding from the radial artery stops.

## After PCI

After PCI, you'll need periodic check-ups and blood tests to monitor your progress. You'll continue to take antiplatelet medication for months or years, and be warned that stopping it early may be deadly. Regardless of your baseline cholesterol level, you also will be started on a statin drug to reduce the risk of a heart attack or death from cardiac causes. Cleveland Clinic cardiologists prescribe a statin to almost every patient who has PCI.

Though cardiac rehabilitation is essential to a full recovery for patients who have had a heart attack or a cardiac stenting procedure, it's estimated that less than 30 percent of patients take advantage of these valuable programs. Cardiac rehabilitation reduces the risk of death, heart attack, and repeat hospitalization by 30 percent.

## Coronary Artery Bypass Grafting (CABG)

Despite the success and popularity of stenting, coronary artery bypass grafting (CABG) remains one of the most frequently performed operations in this country. In certain patient populations, such as diabetics with reduced heart pumping function, CABG reduces the risk of death, compared with PCI.

CABG was pioneered in 1967 by Cleveland Clinic cardiac surgeon Rene G. Favaloro, MD, who took a vein from a patient's leg and used it to successfully reroute oxygen-rich blood around a blockage in the patient's coronary artery. The technique had been tried before, but because surgeons could only guess where the blockages were located, the procedure was largely unsuccessful. The development of

selective coronary angiography by Cleveland Clinic cardiologist Mason Sones, Jr., MD, provided a road map that enabled Dr. Favaloro and other heart surgeons to locate the blockages and reroute blood flow around them.

## What to Expect

CABG is performed exclusively by cardiac and cardiothoracic (heart and lung) surgeons. In the traditional procedure, an incision is made down the middle of the chest, the breastbone (sternum) is split lengthwise, and the ribs are spread apart to provide easy access to the heart. A heart-lung machine is connected to divert the flow of blood from the heart and take over the job of the heart and lungs. This allows the heart to be stopped to make the surgeon's job easier.

In the recommended bypass operation, one end of the left internal thoracic artery (LITA), located on the inside of the chest wall, is sewn to the left anterior descending artery, the most important coronary artery. This reroutes blood around the blockage.

If more than one bypass is needed, the radial artery taken from the arm, or the right ITA should be used (see "Radial Artery Shines as a Second Bypass Graft"). Many surgeons still perform an older procedure using the saphenous vein from the leg. However, the saphenous vein tends to occlude with plaque so quickly that it becomes blocked in 6 to 8 percent of patients before they leave the hospital. Within 10 years, virtually all saphenous vein grafts need to be replaced in another CABG operation. On the other hand, the radial artery usually remains plaque-free indefinitely.

After performing the bypasses, doctors stimulate the heart to start it beating again, take the patient off the heart-lung machine, reconnect the breastbone (sternum), and close the chest.

After CABG, patients usually stay in the hospital for about a week. Recovery generally takes six to eight weeks,

NEW FINDING

### Radial Artery Shines as a Second Bypass Graft

The gold standard for coronary artery bypass grafting (CABG) is attaching the left internal thoracic artery (LITA) to the left anterior descending artery, the heart's most important artery. But when more than one bypass is needed, most surgeons use a vein from the leg. But that may soon change. In 2018, researchers examined six studies comparing CABG operations using the saphenous leg vein to those using the radial artery from the arm, and the radial artery won hands down. When radial artery grafts were used in addition to the LITA, the grafts stayed open longer, and patients were significantly less likely to suffer a heart attack or need another revascularization than when the saphenous vein was used. Use of the radial artery as a second bypass graft reduced the combination outcome of death, heart attack, and revascularization by 33 percent over saphenous veins. Revascularizations alone fell by 50 percent and heart attacks by about 30 percent. Complications were especially low in patients younger than age 75 or with good kidney function, and in women.

*New England Journal of Medicine,* May 31, 2018

although some people may return to normal activities more quickly. Patients at low risk of another heart attack or cardiac death may safely return to normal activity, including work, after only two weeks of recovery.

The good news is that CABG is a relatively safe choice: The expected mortality rate for elective bypass surgery in patients under age 65 without heart failure or a poorly functioning left ventricle is less than one percent—slightly higher in older patients and women. Long-term survival rates are very good, particularly when the LITA and radial artery are used as bypass grafts. Long-term survival may be improved by taking statins prior to the surgery.

## Making CABG More Patient-Friendly

Relatively recent innovations have made CABG easier on patients and possible in high-risk patients.

## Off-Pump Surgery

In older and sicker patients, many surgeons feel that avoiding the heart-lung machine by conducting "off-pump" surgery is safer than using it. In the off-pump procedure, the surgeon performs CABG while the heart is still beating. In the on-pump procedure, the patient's heart is stopped and the surgeon performs the bypass. The blood circulates through the heart-lung machine where it is oxygenated and pumped back into the patient. After the bypass is completed, the heart is restarted.

Randomized clinical trials have shown no difference in outcomes between off-pump and on-pump surgery in high-volume centers. Results have not been as good in centers with less experience. The current thinking is to perform off-pump surgery when the choice is best for the patient, rather than making it the default procedure for CABG.

## Coronary Artery Bypass Grafting (CABG)

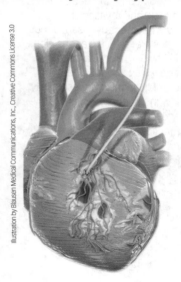 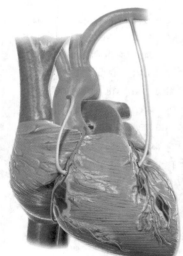 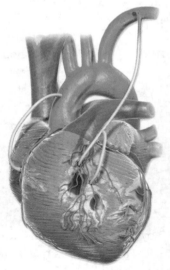 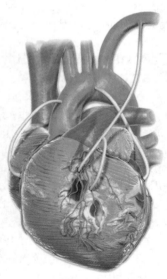

*Illustration by Blausen Medical Communications, Inc., Creative Commons License 3.0*

| Single bypass | Double bypass | Triple bypass | Quadruple bypass |

Coronary artery bypass grafting (CABG) is a surgical procedure used to improve blood flow in arteries of the heart that have become blocked by plaque. In CABG, a healthy artery or vein from elsewhere in the body is sewn to the blocked artery, creating a bypass for blood to flow around the blockage.

If the blockage is isolated in one coronary artery, a single bypass is done. But if there are multiple blockages in more than one artery, a double, triple, or quadruple bypass may be necessary.

## Minimally Invasive Surgery

In January 1996, Cleveland Clinic heart surgeon Delos M. Cosgrove, MD, became the first to operate on an aortic valve without opening the patient's chest. Instead, he made a two-inch incision between the ribs to access the heart and successfully replaced the valve. The patient left the hospital three days later without requiring any pain medication.

This technically difficult approach is now used when a single bypass to the left anterior descending (LAD) artery on the front of the heart is required. Today, the procedure is universally performed with the help of a robot. Advantages of this less-invasive approach include shorter hospital stay, less postoperative pain, less likelihood of needing a blood transfusion, fewer complications, and better cosmetic outcome. However, the minimally invasive approach takes longer to perform, costs more, leaves some patients with inadequate revascularization, and can increase the risk of death.

## Hybrid Revascularizations

In some patients, it is considered reasonable to perform CABG on the LAD and PCI on the remaining vessels. This type of hybrid operation is done in a single procedure requiring only one anesthesia. The dual approach may help prevent complications in patients who would be at higher risk for traditional CABG surgery due to age or the severity and location of their CAD.

## Reducing Postoperative Complications

Atrial fibrillation (AF)—an irregular rhythm or fluttering of the heart's two upper chambers—occurs after heart surgery in about one-third of patients, and can trigger a stroke. Anti-arrhythmia medications and procedures can help avoid this complication.

Another common postoperative complication is pericarditis, or inflammation of the sac around the heart. This painful condition often can be prevented with a nonsteroidal anti-inflammatory drug, such as aspirin or ibuprofen, plus colchicine.

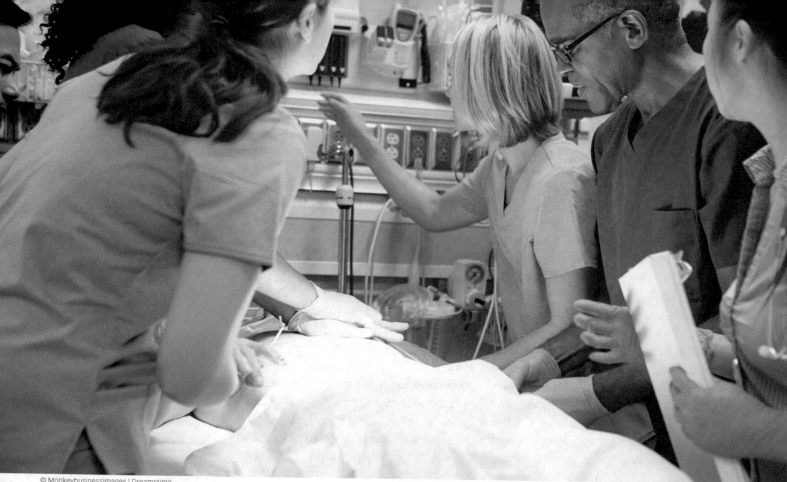

A heart attack is a medical emergency. The sooner treatment begins, the less damage to the heart will occur.

## 7 If You Have A Heart Attack

A heart attack (myocardial infarction, or MI) occurs when a coronary artery suddenly becomes blocked, stopping or severely restricting the flow of blood. When the area of the heart muscle or myocardium relying on this artery is deprived of oxygen for more than a few minutes, all or part of it can die. Immediate treatment is critical. The sooner the flow of oxygenated blood can be restored, the better your chance of recovering, and the better the outcome will be. Half of all patients who die from a heart attack do so within one hour of the first symptoms. After six hours, damage to the myocardium is usually permanent and irreversible, although opening a blocked artery six or more hours after the first symptoms can sometimes be successful. This is why it's very important for you to know the symptoms of a heart attack and what to do if you think you are having a heart attack.

Unfortunately, about one-fifth of heart attack victims have no symptoms, or have very mild symptoms they attribute to indigestion or a flu-like illness. As a result, they don't know they've had a heart attack. The damage to the heart is usually discovered in an ECG taken during a routine physical exam or an exercise stress test. This is known as a silent heart attack.

### Encouraging Numbers

Fortunately, efforts to improve heart attack survival are working: Deaths from heart attack continue to drop (see "More Women Surviving Heart Attacks, on page 59").

### Location Determines Prognosis

Survival after a heart attack depends partly on what part of the heart muscle is affected and how much of it dies. Blockages that occur in the main artery on the front of the heart (left anterior descending artery) can be deadly, especially when they occur in the first one-third of the vessel. If 30 to 40 percent of the heart muscle is injured, or the left ventricle is severely injured, the heart will no longer be able to pump effectively, and the prognosis is likely to be worse.

Aggressive treatment with medical therapy and early angioplasty or CABG has been shown to prevent more deaths or heart attacks than medical therapy alone. Similarly, aggressive medical treatment and preventive measures in patients with angina, heart rhythm disturbances, or heart failure lowers the risk of another heart attack or death.

During a heart attack, cardiologists say that "time is myocardium," and treatment is geared toward quickly restoring blood flow to the compromised heart muscle tissue. This can be achieved with stenting or, less often today, with drugs to dissolve the blood clot. Once you are stable, your cardiologist can determine whether CABG, further stenting, or medical therapy is the best approach to keep the coronary arteries open and prevent another heart attack. This may require your transfer to a hospital with more experience treating heart patients.

## Emergency Treatment

One of the first things an emergency room physician or EMT must do is confirm that you are having a heart attack. Any patient with symptoms of a heart attack is diagnosed with acute coronary syndrome (ACS). An ECG and blood samples will help determine if the heart has been injured and, if so, how severely.

Sometimes, the clinical signs and symptoms together with the ECG recording indicate that treatment must begin immediately. Although much progress has been made to identify high-risk patients, low-risk patients still pose a diagnostic challenge for physicians. Although some studies of coronary CT angiography (CTA) have confirmed the value of this noninvasive technology for determining which patients with chest pain may be safely sent home, other studies have found that CTA was more likely to lead to hospital admission and angiography. Cleveland Clinic does not use CTA alone to rule out heart attack, but may use CTA in conjunction with other tests to rule out heart attack in low-risk patients.

## Improved Treatment Guidelines for STEMI Patients

The type of heart attack known as an ST-elevation myocardial infarction (STEMI) occurs when a plaque ruptures in a coronary artery, creating a clot that completely obstructs blood flow. A large area of the heart potentially may be affected. Complications can include death, heart failure, or a heart rhythm abnormality that can lead to cardiac arrest.

Treatment guidelines focus on clinical decision-making at all stages, beginning with the onset of symptoms at home or work, systems of care to ensure that patients get immediate treatment, and the rapid restoration of blood flow down the obstructed coronary artery. When there are delays, which may occur when a patient arrives at a hospital where PCI is not performed, clot-busting drugs should be administered, if safe for the individual patient. The patient should then be transferred to a facility where PCI can subsequently be performed, if needed.

## Primary PCI

Until recently, clots that block the coronary arteries were dissolved with thrombolytic agents given intravenously. But the risk of bleeding in the brain is lower with PCI than with thrombolytic drugs, and when the procedure can be performed rapidly, it is more effective in reducing the risk of recurrent heart attack or death.

Today at Cleveland Clinic and other medical centers with around-the-clock cath labs, all patients with STEMI, are taken directly from the ambulance to the cath lab for PCI, avoiding the emergency department altogether. This helps ensure the artery is opened within the

**NEW FINDING**

### More Women Surviving Heart Attacks

The number of women who die in the hospital following a full-blown heart attack dropped from 18.3 percent to 6.9 percent over the past two decades. The news was equally good for women who suffered a mild heart attack: Their in-hospital morality rate fell from 11 percent to 3.6 percent. The death rate in men also declined, but less dramatically. The researchers involved in this 50,000-patient study theorized that the significant increase in survival rate for women is likely due to improvement in their heart attacks being recognized, taken seriously and treated appropriately.

*European Society of Cardiology* 2017 Congress

## The Symptoms of a Heart Attack

If you think all heart attacks will cause you to clutch your chest and drop to the floor, you may have seen too many movies. Although this type of dramatic pain and collapse can occur, symptoms of heart attack are frequently far more subtle and can vary widely, especially in women, people with diabetes, and older adults.

### Men

During a heart attack, men tend to experience:

- Chest pressure growing in frequency and intensity over two to three days (unstable angina) and often described as a squeezing sensation
- Pain in the left arm, shoulder, neck, or jaw that may or may not stem from pain in the center of the chest. It also may occur in the right arm
- Pain in the abdomen that may be mistaken for indigestion
- Sweating, restlessness, and anxiety
- Dizziness, faintness, and heavy pounding in the chest
- Shortness of breath
- Disorientation (more common in the elderly)
- Nausea or queasiness (more common in women)

### Women

During a heart attack, women may experience the same symptoms as men, However, they tend to experience symptoms that are less dramatic and are frequently mistaken for less-serious conditions.

A woman who experiences any of the following symptoms should seek immediate medical attention:

- Upper back or shoulder pain
- Jaw pain or pain that radiates to the jaw
- Pain that radiates to the arm
- Pressure or pain in the center of the chest
- Nausea or queasiness and indigestion
- Shortness of breath or feeling "winded"
- Unusual fatigue for several days
- Lightheadedness

## What to Do if You Suspect a Heart Attack

If you may be having a heart attack, it is better to be safe than sorry.

- If symptoms last 15 minutes, call 911 for an ambulance.
- Do not delay, and do not attempt to drive to the hospital.
- The sooner you get to the hospital, the easier it will be to treat you. The longer you wait, the greater your chance of dying or suffering extensive damage.

**Take the following steps:**

- Tell your concerns to the people around you, or make a quick phone call to a relative or close friend.
- Sit or lie down.
- If you have nitroglycerin tablets, take one under the tongue every five minutes, up to a total of three pills.
- If you do not have nitroglycerin, chew an adult-sized (325 mg) aspirin.
- Remember to call 911, as outlined above.

recommended 90-minute window. In fact, Cleveland Clinic's enhanced protocol for treating STEMI patients has slashed this time to an average of 52 minutes and as little as 21 minutes. These quicker revascularizations result in fewer deaths and better quality of life for survivors.

At smaller and more remote hospitals, thrombolytic therapy may still be used with good results. However, when a patient does not get relief from thrombolytic therapy quickly, the cardiologist will perform emergency or "rescue" PCI. Although the optimal timing of intervention has not yet been determined, there is overwhelming evidence that taking action instead of waiting saves lives. The risk of death increases for every 30 minutes that elapses before a patient with STEMI is treated.

In some patients, an intra-aortic balloon pump, Impella, or extra-corporeal membrane oxygenation (ECMO) may be used to reduce the work of the heart and increase coronary artery blood flow while preparations for PCI begin. This tends to help stabilize dangerously low blood pressure and prevent cardiogenic shock, which can cause organs to fail when they don't get the blood supply they need. Shock is a very serious, often fatal, situation that is difficult to reverse. Nevertheless, the combination of intra-aortic balloon pump and rescue stenting enables many of these patients to survive a heart attack.

## Recovery

Recovery from heart attack depends on a variety of factors, including the severity of the disease, how much heart muscle was affected, how fast blood flow was restored, and the patient's overall health and fitness. This is one case where carrying a little extra weight may be valuable, even lifesaving. Patients with low body weight who suffer a heart attack are at increased risk of dying, possibly because the absence of physiological reserve and fat stores hinder the ability to handle the stresses of a heart attack.

Complete recovery is possible after a heart attack—even a severe one—when it is treated quickly. Even a mild heart attack can cause permanent injury and hinder recovery if it is not promptly treated. The greater the proportion of the heart affected by a heart attack, the greater the risk of developing heart failure. But no matter the extent of injury, it is important to do everything you can to prevent another heart attack, sudden cardiac death, or heart failure after you are discharged from the hospital. This includes exercising to strengthen your heart muscle and seeking treatment if you are depressed.

## Preventing a Second Heart Attack

The drugs that you start taking and lifestyle changes you make after your first heart attack to prevent another are called secondary prevention measures.

If your heart attack was caused by a blood clot, your doctor may prescribe a combination of medications that includes aspirin; clopidogrel (Plavix®), ticagrelor (Brilinta®), or prasugrel (Effient®); a statin; and a beta blocker to reduce your chance of dying from heart disease or needing bypass surgery. You also may be prescribed an ACE inhibitor or ARB. Patients who take proton-pump inhibitors (PPIs) such as omeprazole (Prilosec®) or esomeprazole (Nexium®) to reduce gastric acid production should be aware that PPIs may interfere with the beneficial effects of clopidogrel.

It also is recommended that patients:

- **Undergoing an invasive procedure receive aspirin plus another antiplatelet medication;**

- **Take ticagrelor or clopidogrel,** whether they are being treated with medical therapy alone or also are having an invasive procedure;

- **Undergoing medical treatment alone take aspirin indefinitely and clopidogrel or ticagrelor for at least 12 months.**

It is absolutely necessary to take all your medications as prescribed and never stop taking them without your doctor's permission (see "Stopping Low-Dose Aspirin Ups Heart-Attack and Stroke Risk"). Studies have shown that people who do not fill their prescriptions after suffering a heart attack are far more likely to die within a year than those who fill their prescriptions and take the medications as prescribed. If you experience any type of side effects from the drugs you are taking, contact your doctor right away.

Your doctor will want to review your risk factors with you. It is up to you to do all you can to eliminate them to prevent a second heart attack. Remember that having a heart attack puts you at risk for having another one. The second one is likely to occur in a different location or a different artery than your first heart attack. This underscores the need to make lifestyle changes and take medications designed to reverse atherosclerosis or prevent it from getting worse.

## Preventing Sudden Cardiac Death

Sudden cardiac death (SCD)—also called cardiac arrest—occurs when the heart stops working abruptly and without warning. Cardiac arrest can happen to people who appear to be completely healthy, but it is about four to six times more likely to happen to people who survived a heart attack. Sudden cardiac death is not always sudden or "out of the blue." Studies in which family members or bystanders were interviewed suggest that up to 80 percent of patients had symptoms that lasted up to several hours and were either misunderstood or ignored.

The risk of sudden cardiac death is highest in the first 30 days after a heart attack

## Implantable Cardioverter-Defibrillator

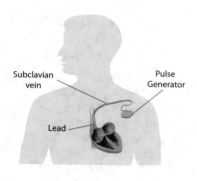

Subclavian vein

Pulse Generator

Lead

**Single chamber**

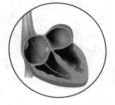

**Dual chamber**

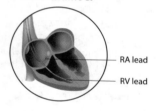

RA lead

RV lead

**Biventricular**

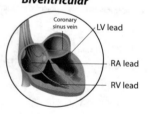

Coronary sinus vein

LV lead

RA lead

RV lead

© AliiaO7 | Dreamstime

An implantable cardioverter-defibrillator (ICD) is placed under the skin, often near the left collarbone. The leads (wires that conduct electricity) may be threaded into the left subclavian vein (which returns blood to the heart from the left arm) all the way into the right ventricle. Or they are placed on the surface of the heart. Leads placed into the vein do not interfere with blood flow.

and is most likely to affect patients with a left ventricular ejection fraction of less than 40 percent. The risk drops continually over a two-year period.

Cardiac arrest is not synonymous with heart attack, because it does not require blood flow through the coronary arteries to be blocked. Rather, cardiac arrest is a malfunction of the heart's electrical system that prevents it from contracting properly. Nevertheless, coronary artery blockages are one important cause of cardiac arrest.

The heart contains specialized fibers that conduct electrical impulses from its own pacemaker throughout the heart muscle in a well-coordinated fashion. These impulses are timed to make the heart muscle contract in a way that pumps blood effectively, squeezing it from the bottom to the top, where the main arteries leave the heart. The most common heart rhythm disorder (arrhythmia) causing cardiac arrest is ventricular fibrillation (VF). During VF, the electrical impulses spread randomly throughout the heart, making the heart muscle quiver (fibrillate). It becomes unable to produce a contraction forceful enough to eject blood. The brain is the first to suffer the effects of absent blood flow, so loss of consciousness occurs within seconds.

Treatment must begin within minutes, or serious brain injury or death results. Shocking the heart with a defibrillator can stop the random electrical impulses flowing through it. Ideally, the heart's natural pacemaker will then start up by itself, sending its electrical impulses down the proper paths and restoring the heart's normal rhythm. While waiting for a defibrillator to arrive, the victim of cardiac arrest must receive CPR, or damage to vital organs will inevitably occur.

If you've had a heart attack, you are at an increased risk of cardiac arrest. Your odds of experiencing cardiac arrest increase if you have a poorly functioning heart (low ejection fraction) that leaves behind an abnormally large proportion of blood in its ventricles after a heartbeat.

In general, the larger and more serious your heart attack, the more likely you'll end up with a poorly functioning heart with a low ejection fraction and/or arrhythmia, even after emergency PCI or CABG.

After you have recovered from a heart attack, your cardiologist will tell you if you are at increased risk of cardiac arrest and will discuss treatment options. Beta blockers may help you maintain a normal heart rhythm and prevent arrhythmias. New evidence indicates that omega-3 fatty acids, which are found naturally in ocean fish and in supplement form, may help protect against sudden cardiac death. However, the most effective treatment known to date is an implantable cardioverter-defibrillator (ICD).

### Device Therapy

Your cardiologist may decide that you would benefit from an ICD, an electronic device that monitors your heart rhythm and delivers a shock when it detects a rapid, disorganized heart rhythm, such as ventricular fibrillation or ventricular tachycardia. Most ICDs also act as a pacemaker if your heart rhythm becomes dangerously slow or irregular. An ICD is recommended if your ejection fraction (heart pumping function) is 35 percent or less (a normal ejection fraction is 55 to 65 percent). As several clinical trials demonstrated, there is a significant decrease in the risk of death in patients who receive an ICD after a heart attack.

ICDs have become increasingly popular as miniaturization and computer technologies have downsized these devices to the point where they can be placed under the skin, usually near the collarbone, without causing any discomfort. The newest ICDs are implanted in a procedure similar to cardiac catheterization and immediately tested to ensure they work properly.

ICDs work by continually monitoring your heart rate and recognizing any arrhythmias that occur. If an ICD detects ventricular tachycardia or fibrillation, it will first try to correct the rhythm by "pacing" the heart with a burst of electrical impulses. If this works, the ICD will return to its monitoring mode. If not, it will send a more powerful electrical shock to the heart. Patients say it feels like a thump on the chest.

ICD batteries last four to eight years, depending on how many times the device "kicks in." An ICD must be replaced when its battery runs down.

## Heart Failure

After a heart attack, some patients find that their heart doesn't completely recover, and they are unable to resume normal activities without becoming fatigued or out of breath. These are the first signs of heart failure. The heart attack may have caused some of the individual heart muscle cells to die. Over time, these permanently damaged areas of the heart become thinned and useless, or scarred and stiff. Either way, the heart no longer can pump as efficiently as it did before and is unable to meet the body's demand for oxygenated blood.

Heart failure also can occur from high blood pressure, valve disease, or diseases that attack the heart muscle. Diabetes increases the risk, as do certain chemotherapy agents.

Heart failure often occurs gradually. In an effort to do its job, the heart undergoes a series of compensatory changes called "remodeling," which are actually destructive. Remodeling is a vicious cycle. The weaker the heart becomes, the harder it tries to compensate for its inability to pump, and the less likely it is able to do so. In its early stages, heart failure may not produce many symptoms. As it progresses, patients may experience some disturbing symptoms (see "How Heart Failure Can Affect Memory"). While the number and type of symptoms may vary from patient to patient, the primary symptoms are shortness of breath, fatigue, and fluid retention.

Preventing heart failure, or managing it when you get it, is a complex process that usually requires diet, exercise, and other lifestyle changes, as well as the use of many medications. When bypass surgery or valve surgery can be used to restore blood flow to viable heart tissue, the treatment may actually reverse heart failure. Some patients require a new mechanical device to boost their heart's pumping power.

Treatment is always individualized. The priorities are finding ways to help the heart pump more efficiently, relieving symptoms, and preventing the left ventricle—the heart's main pumping chamber—from growing larger and weaker. Today, many medical and surgical treatment options are available, allowing greater numbers of patients to prevent or delay the onset of heart failure after a heart attack. More effective medications and sophisticated new surgical approaches are helping patients with the condition live longer and more normal lives.

## Heart Failure Is a Progressive Disease

Heart failure is traditionally classified by how well patients can perform normal activities of daily life. Doctors call this "functional capacity." The New York Heart Association (NYHA) functional classification is the most widely used system. Most cases of mild and moderate heart failure can be treated to prevent heart failure from progressing. Most patients' symptoms will improve if they are treated appropriately and risk factors are eliminated.

## NYHA Classification of Heart Failure Severity

### Class I (No Impairment)

Patients have heart disease but without resulting limitation of physical activity. Ordinary physical activity does not cause undue fatigue, palpitation, dyspnea (shortness of breath), or anginal pain (chest, jaw or arm discomfort).

### Class II (Mild to Moderate)

Patients have heart disease resulting in slight limitation of physical activity. They are comfortable at rest. Ordinary physical activity results in fatigue, palpitation, dyspnea, or anginal pain (chest, jaw or arm discomfort).

### How Heart Failure Can Affect Memory

The brain is highly dependent on a steady flow of oxygenated blood. When the heart is unable to meet the brain's needs—for example, when heart failure weakens the heart's pumping power—brain function is impaired.

When a group of 314 healthy participants underwent MRI brain scans, those with reduced cardiac output showed less blood flow to the left and right temporal lobes—areas responsible for memory processing and the location where Alzheimer's disease starts. These findings reinforce that raising cardiac output with exercise and medications helps maintain brain health, as well as heart health. Increasing cardiac output also may help prevent early memory loss from progressing.

*Neurology*, online Nov. 8, 2017

### Drug Makes Breast Cancer Treatment Safer for the Heart

Chemotherapy agents called anthracyclines save the lives of countless women with breast cancer, only to cause heart failure later. But the angiotensin-receptor blocker (ARB) candesartan (Atacand®) may help preserve the heart's function. In 2015, researchers discovered that candesartan taken daily starting in the early stages of cancer treatment helped preserve the heart's pumping power as measured by left ventricular ejection fraction. Although the clinical trial was small, the finding brings hope for women who need lifesaving chemotherapy.

### Class III (Moderate)

Patients have cardiac disease resulting in marked limitation of physical activity. They are comfortable at rest. Less-than-ordinary physical activity results in fatigue, palpitation, dyspnea, or anginal pain (chest, jaw or arm discomfort).

### Class IV (Severe)

Patients have cardiac disease resulting in inability to carry on any physical activity. Symptoms of heart failure or angina may be present even at rest. If any physical activity is undertaken, symptoms worsen.

## ACC/AHA Classification System and Recommended Therapy

The American College of Cardiology (ACC) and the American Heart Association (AHA) classify heart failure based on the progression of the disease. The ACC/AHA classification includes patients at risk for developing heart failure, and those who have structural heart disease but no symptoms.

This classification system was created because the NYHA system is a subjective assessment made by a physician that represents a patient's condition at the time of evaluation. A patient's NYHA class may change between visits as treatments take effect or the disease progresses. In contrast, the ACC/AHA system classifies patients objectively based on disease progression and structural changes in the heart. Each stage is linked to treatments that are uniquely appropriate for that stage. Only ACC/AHA stages B, C, and D are comparable to the NYHA classification system. There is no NYHA class comparable to stage A.

### Stage A

Patients are at high risk for developing heart failure but have no structural disorder of the heart. Patients at this stage have no symptoms. Treatment is focused on eliminating or reducing risk factors through lifestyle modifications, such as diet, exercise, and avoidance of tobacco, illicit drugs, and excessive alcohol. Hypertension, diabetes, or high blood cholesterol levels should be treated appropriately. Additionally, patients with diabetes and/or confirmed coronary artery disease should be prescribed an ACE inhibitor or ARB, cholesterol-lowering drugs (statins), and/or aspirin.

### Stage B

Patients have no apparent symptoms of heart failure, but confirmed structural heart disease. Most have suffered a recent heart attack in which left ventricular function was largely preserved. Others have cardiomyopathy or valve disease. In addition to the lifestyle modifications and medications listed for stage A, most patients should take an ACE inhibitor (or ARB) and beta blockers. An implantable defibrillator may be advised in selected patients with low ejection fraction.

### Stage C

Patients have structural heart disease and symptoms of heart failure, such as shortness of breath, fatigue, and reduced exercise tolerance. In addition to all measures appropriate for stages A and B, they should restrict salt intake, use a diuretic, and take an ACE inhibitor or ARB and a beta blocker, or an angiotensin receptor-neprilysin inhibitor (ARNI). Some may derive symptomatic benefit from digoxin, but this drug does not prolong life. An aldosterone blocker, such as spironolactone (Aldactone®) or eplerenone (Inspra®), may be prescribed for left ventricular dysfunction following a heart attack. If heart failure progresses, surgical intervention should be considered. In late stage C (comparable to NYHA class III or IV heart failure), an aldosterone blocker may be advised. An implantable defibrillator is recommended for all patients with a left ventricular ejection fraction of less than 35 percent. Some patients may be eligible for cardiac resynchronization therapy (described later in this chapter).

### Stage D

Patients are severely ill and require special medical and/or surgical intervention.

Intravenous diuretics and vasodilators may be appropriate for hospitalized patients. These patients may be considered for a heart transplant, ventricular assist device (VAD), or an investigational surgery or drugs. End-stage patients who are not eligible for any of these extraordinary procedures may be referred for hospice care.

## Medical Therapy for Heart Failure

Over the past few decades, standard medical therapy for heart failure has gradually evolved into a sophisticated combination of treatments that changes as the condition progresses. The most effective medications and dosages for each patient vary widely.

It is common for heart failure patients to require medications for other diseases as well—for example, diabetes. It is very important that your doctor knows what other drugs you are taking, as your heart failure medications may interact with them and cause side effects. They may even make your symptoms worse.

## Standard Medications for Heart Failure

### ACE Inhibitors

Until ACE inhibitors were developed, the diagnosis of heart failure came with a very short life expectancy. That is no longer the case. ACE inhibitors are a major contributor to the improved prognosis for heart failure patients who receive treatment early in the development of their condition.

ACE inhibitors work by dilating blood vessels, allowing blood to flow more easily. This makes it easier for the heart to pump blood out to the body. Originally developed as a medication for high blood pressure, ACE inhibitors are now known to do much more. ACE inhibitors reduce heart rate, decrease the incidence of sudden death and heart attack, improve quality of life, enhance blood flow to the kidneys, improve sodium excretion, increase exercise tolerance, and prevent and perhaps even reverse detrimental remodeling. ACE inhibitors are considered to be an essential component of medical therapy for the treatment of heart failure.

## Medications Commonly Used in the Treatment of Heart Failure

| TYPE OF DRUG | WHAT IT DOES |
| --- | --- |
| Aldosterone blockers | Blocks the harmful effects of aldosterone in patients with severe heart failure. |
| Anticoagulants and antiplatelet agents | Prevents the formation of potentially harmful blood clots, especially in heart failure patients with atrial fibrillation, by decreasing the ability of platelets to stick together and form clots. |
| Angiotensin-converting enzyme (ACE) inhibitors | Dilates blood vessels to reduce blood pressure, improves the heart's output of blood, and increases blood flow to the kidneys. ACE inhibitors also block the production of angiotensin II. |
| Angiotensin receptor blocker (ARBs) | ARBs have the same effects as ACE inhibitors. |
| Angiotensin receptor/neprilysin inhibitors (ARNIs) | Relaxes blood vessels and eliminates excess fluid and sodium. |
| Anti-arrhythmic agents | Controls the heart's rhythm and helps prevent irregular rhythms. |
| Beta blockers | Slows the heart rate, decreases the force of contraction, and reduces blood pressure. By blocking the "beta-adrenergic receptors" of the heart, it blocks the detrimental actions of excess epinephrine (adrenaline) and norepinephrine (noradrenaline) on heart muscle. |
| Digoxin | Improves the heart's pumping ability and lowers high levels of neurohormones, which aggravate heart failure. |
| Diuretics | Removes extra fluid from the tissues and bloodstream, lessens edema (swelling), and makes breathing easier. |
| Inotropic agent | Improves the heart's pumping function and raises blood pressure in patients with cardiac shock or low cardiac output. |
| Potassium and magnesium | Replaces electrolytes lost with increased urination when taking certain diuretics. |
| Vasodilators Hydralazine/nitrate | Dilates (opens) the arteries and veins. |

## Angiotensin II Receptor Blockers

Not everyone can tolerate ACE inhibitors. If they produce an intolerable cough, dizziness, distortion in the sense of taste, or swelling of the face and throat, an angiotensin receptor blocker (ARB) may be an acceptable substitute.

The effects of ARBs and ACE inhibitors are similar, but ARBs are less likely to produce a cough. No ARB is superior to ACE inhibitors, but if you have heart failure with a low ejection fraction and cannot tolerate ACE inhibitors, taking an ARB in addition to other medications is better than not taking an ARB at all. If you have heart failure with preserved systolic function, taking an ARB in addition to other medications may help keep you out of the hospital.

## ARNIs

Cardiologists consider a new class of drugs called angiotensin receptor/neprilysin inhibitors (ARNIs) to be one of the most exciting developments in heart failure in decades. The drug relaxes blood vessels and eliminates excess fluid and sodium in an entirely new way. In clinical trials, the first drug in this class, sacubitril/valsartan (Entresto®) showed dramatic ability to reduce deaths and hospitalizations in patients with heart failure, while improving their quality of life (see "New Heart Failure Drug Improves Quality of Life"). Its benefits were so striking that the FDA expedited approval of the drug. ARNIs are now recommended as a replacement for ACE inhibitors and ARBs in patients with NYHA II and III heart failure and an ejection fraction less than 35 percent to further lower hospitalizations and mortality.

## Beta Blockers

Although beta blockers were widely used for years to treat hypertension, their ability to make the heart beat less forcefully and more slowly was assumed to be harmful to patients with heart failure. But in reality, beta blockers can be extremely helpful in improving the heart's pumping ability. Studies showed that patients taking beta blockers had up to 50 percent fewer deaths from fatal heart attack. Beta blockers were also found to slow the progression of heart failure, improve NYHA functional class, and reduce the risk of hospitalization. They may also prevent many of the harmful effects of ventricular remodeling and arrhythmias that occur with heart failure. With respect to remodeling, beta blockers can increase the ejection fraction and reduce the size of the heart. These biologic effects appear to reverse remodeling and return the heart toward normal.

Two beta blockers have been approved for use in heart failure: carvedilol (Coreg® and Coreg CR®) and extended-release metoprolol (Toprol XL®). Their most common side effects are dizziness, slow heart beat (bradycardia), shortness of breath, and fatigue. These side effects usually can be managed by adjusting the dose.

---

## Drugs to Avoid if You Have Heart Failure

These drugs should not be used, or should be used with extreme caution, by patients with heart failure.

**Calcium channel blockers**

- Nifedipine (Adalat®, Procardia®)
- Diltiazem (Cardizem®)
- Verapamil (Calan®)

**Anti-arrhythmics**

- Flecainide (Tambocor®)
- Propafenone (Rythmol®)
- Disopyramide (Norpace®)
- Quinidine (Quinidex®)
- Procainamide (Procanbid®)
- Sotalol (Betapace®)
- Dronedarone (Multaq®)

**TZD anti-diabetic agents (thiazolidinediones)**

- Pioglitazone (Actos®)

**Tricyclic antidepressants**

- Desipramine (Norpramin®)
- Protriptyline (Vivactil®)

- Amitriptyline (Elavil®)
- Nortriptyline (Pamelor®, Aventyl®)

**Nonsteroidal anti-inflammatory drugs (NSAIDs)**

- Ibuprofen (Advil®, Motrin®)
- Diclofenac (Cataflam®, Voltaren®)
- Celecoxib (Celebrex®)
- Sulindac (Clinoril®)
- Indomethacin (Indocin®)
- Naproxen (Aleve®, Naprosyn®)

**Decongestants**

- Ephedrine (Sudafed®)

**DPP-4 inhibitors**

- Saxagliptin (Onglyza®)
- Saxagliptin plus metformin extended release (Kombiglyze XR®)
- Alogliptin (Nesina®)
- Alogliptin plus metformin (Kazano®)
- Alogliptin plus pioglitazone (Oseni®)

---

Patients with decompensated heart failure or fluid retention should not use beta blockers. Patients with severe diabetes, asthma, or peripheral vascular disease may not be able to tolerate beta blockers.

## Diuretics

Drugs that rid the body of excess sodium and water are called diuretics. Diuretics are used in heart failure to decrease swelling and relieve shortness of breath. Several varieties of diuretics exist, but the main type used in heart failure is the loop diuretic, which owes its name to the part of the kidney it acts upon (the Loop of Henle). Drugs in this class include furosemide (Lasix®), torsemide (Demadex®), bumetanide (Bumex®), and ethacrynic acid (Edecrin®).

Heart failure specialists prescribe loop diuretics for 90 percent of heart failure patients, but they strive to use the lowest effective dose. A few patients with mild or moderate heart failure taking an ACE inhibitor and beta blocker may not require diuretics. As heart failure becomes more severe, diuretic requirements often increase.

## Digoxin

Digoxin helps the weakened heart contract more strongly. Clinical trials have shown that digoxin can improve symptoms, functional capacity, exercise tolerance, and quality of life in patients with heart failure. In general, however, digoxin has no effect on survival.

Women, elderly adults, and people with kidney failure are more likely to suffer toxic effects from digoxin and must use it with caution. However, digoxin does appear to reduce heart failure-related hospitalizations, especially in patients with a very low ejection fraction (25 percent or less), so it continues to have a role in the heart-failure care.

## Aldosterone Antagonists

Spironolactone (Aldactone®) and eplerenone (Inspra®) suppress the action of aldosterone, a hormone that causes the kidneys to retain sodium and water. Extra fluid in the body increases blood volume, which puts unwanted strain on an overworked, poorly functioning heart. In addition to helping eliminate excess water, these drugs have the ability to reverse left ventricular remodeling and improve survival.

Aldosterone can cause gynecomastia (breast enlargement in men). Because eplerenone works differently, it does not cause gynecomastia. Both spironolactone and eplerenone can raise serum potassium levels, so potassium levels must be checked within a week or two of starting the drug. This is especially important for patients with kidney failure, who are more prone to developing high potassium.

## Hydralazine Plus a Nitrate

Nitrates release nitric oxide, which dilates arteries and veins. Hydralazine helps increase the effectiveness of nitrates. Together, they improve hemodynamics, reduce the workload of the heart, lower blood pressure, and relieve symptoms. The combination of hydralazine plus a nitrate (Imdur®, Isordil®, or Nitropatch®) is useful in patients whose kidneys are unable to effectively remove waste or who develop high potassium levels. When either problem is a result of ACE inhibitor use, the combination may be substituted. The combination also is approved as add-on therapy for patients who continue to experience symptoms of class III and class IV heart failure despite therapy with ACE inhibitors, beta blockers, and spironolactone. Finally, African-Americans have been shown to derive particular benefit from the nitrate-hydralazine combination.

## Intravenous Vasodilators

Intravenous therapy with nesiritide, nitroglycerin, or nitroprusside may be given to critically ill patients to dilate arteries and veins.

Nesiritide (Natrecor®) is administered in the hospital or emergency department to patients with decompensated heart failure. Patients are given an initial bolus followed

NEW FINDING

### New Heart-Failure Drug Improves Quality of Life

A new class of drugs known as ARNIs not only reduces deaths and hospitalizations, but also gives heart-failure patients a boost in quality of life.

To date, sacubitril/valsartan (Entresto®) is the only ARNI to receive approval by the U.S. Food & Drug Administration. In a clinical trial of 8,400 patients comparing Entresto with the ACE inhibitor enalapril, patients who received the ARNI reported significantly better scores in most physical and social activities than those who took enalapril. The ARNI improved their ability to walk, jog, garden, and participate in hobbies. The greatest improvements were seen in their ability to do household chores and participate in sexual relationships. Improvements began at 8 months and lasted throughout the 36-month study. The improvement in quality of life was equivalent to rolling back the calendar nine years, the authors said.
*JAMA Cardiology*, online April 4, 2018

by a constant infusion. The initial dose and infusion rate is based on the patient's weight. During infusion, blood pressure is monitored regularly, and the infusion is stopped if blood pressure drops significantly.

Nitroglycerin and nitroprusside are options that can be started in the emergency department and continued in the intensive care unit. Nitroglycerin can be converted to oral medication for use after discharge.

## Intravenous Inotropes

Intravenous inotropes include dobutamine and milrinone. They are used in critically ill heart failure patients with shock, low blood pressure, or low cardiac output. They also are given to patients awaiting a heart transplant and as continuous palliative therapy to improve quality of life for end-stage heart failure patients who wish to remain at home.

Intravenous inotropes are not recommended for routine treatment of acute decompensated heart failure, due to lack of long-term benefit and increased risk of complications such as hypotension (low blood pressure) and arrhythmias. They also tend to increase the risk of death during the period immediately after they are started.

## Other Drugs Used for Heart Failure

### Anti-Arrhythmia Medications

Patients with heart failure can develop heart rhythm abnormalities. One of the most common arrhythmias is atrial fibrillation, which affects up to 30 percent of patients with heart failure. This rapid, constant, unregulated contraction of atrial muscle cells in a disorganized manner prevents the heart from filling properly. Atrial fibrillation causes the ventricles to contract more rapidly, dropping cardiac output up to 20 percent due to the loss of normal rhythm. It also increases the risk of a blood clot (thrombus), which can cause a stroke, peripheral embolism, or pulmonary embolism.

Atrial fibrillation may resolve spontaneously, although it often requires the help of drugs or electric shock (cardioversion). If it

continues to occur, antiarrhythmic agents such as amiodarone (Cordarone®, Pacerone®) or dofetilide (Tikosyn®), or a catheter-based technique called ablation, may be used for prevention or treatment.

Ventricular arrhythmias are known to increase the risk of sudden death. Efforts to suppress these arrhythmias with drug therapy have been disappointing. Surgically implanted defibrillators that control heart rhythm are often recommended and are better than anti-arrhythmic drugs for preventing sudden death.

## Anticoagulants and Antiplatelet Agents

The role of antiplatelet drugs such as aspirin and clopidogrel in heart failure remains unclear. These drugs inhibit the function of platelets—small, circulating blood cells that help form clots. Aspirin, clopidogrel, ticagrelor, and prasugrel significantly reduce the risk of heart attack in patients with coronary artery disease and reduce the risk of death following heart attack. Thus, patients with heart attack and coronary artery disease should definitely take aspirin, and in some cases, clopidogrel, ticagrelor, or prasugrel as well. It is unclear whether these drugs are effective in patients with heart failure who have not had a heart attack or have no evidence of coronary artery disease, as clinical trials have been inconclusive.

Warfarin (Coumadin®) is an anticoagulant given to patients at risk for blood clots. The value of warfarin in uncomplicated heart failure is uncertain. However, if a heart failure patient has experienced atrial fibrillation, either warfarin or a novel oral anticoagulant (NOAC), such as the direct thrombin inhibitor dabigatran (Pradaxa®), or the factor Xa ("10-A") inhibitors apixaban (Eliquis®), edoxaban (Savaysa®), or rivaroxaban (Xarelto®), may be prescribed.

## Potassium and Magnesium Supplements

One risk of diuretic therapy is the depletion of potassium (hypokalemia) and/or magnesium (hypomagnesemia), which increases the likelihood of developing a life-threatening arrhythmia. Fortunately, these conditions are easily corrected with potassium or magnesium supplements. Hypokalemia is less likely to occur in patients taking ACE inhibitors and spironolactone or eplerenone. In fact, as mentioned earlier, the opposite situation—high serum potassium levels—can occur with aldosterone blockers. Patients taking potassium supplements may need to stop or reduce their supplements when starting spironolactone or eplerenone therapy.

### Statins

Although higher cholesterol levels are beneficial for patients with heart failure, these patients actually do better when they take statins. Statins lower cholesterol, reducing heart attacks, and death. But they also have other beneficial effects, including the ability to reduce inflammatory factors and cytokines, improve endothelial function, and stabilize plaque. Patients with heart failure who take statins have a lower risk of death and hospitalization for heart failure than non-statin users.

### Other Drugs

One drug with potential is sildenafil, more commonly known as Viagra®, which also is sold under the name Revatio®. Sildenafil offers a number of benefits in heart failure with pulmonary hypertension; specifically it allows patients to breathe better. It also appears to limit the deterioration process.

## Other Treatment Options for Heart Failure

When medications are insufficient to manage heart failure, other options are available. Bypass surgery or stenting may be used to improve blood flow to the heart muscle. Defective heart valves may be repaired or replaced via surgical procedures. These measures often help the heart regain its ability to pump properly and may even cause the symptoms of heart failure to disappear.

When a large portion of the heart muscle is damaged beyond repair, or the coronary arteries are extensively diseased, exciting electronic devices, mechanical circulatory support systems, and surgical procedures offer hope for these patients.

### Cardiac Resynchronization Therapy (Biventricular Pacing)

In heart failure, interruptions in the electrical pathways in the heart cause the right ventricle to contract at a different rate than the left ventricle. Instead of a smooth, coordinated contraction, this lack of synchronization (dyssynchrony) can reduce the heart's ability to pump blood.

Cardiac resynchronization therapy (CRT) is a method of making the ventricles work together in sync. It involves implanting a pacemaker, usually in the left front chest below the collarbone, and threading three electrodes into the heart through a vein. One is positioned in the right atrium, one in the right ventricle, and one in the left cardiac vein (to stimulate the left ventricle). The electrodes are programmed to stimulate both sides of the heart simultaneously. The frequency and timing are adjusted to optimally coordinate the contraction of the atria and ventricles to produce a more efficient heartbeat. This results in better blood flow, which improves heart failure symptoms and quality of life and reduces complications and risk of death. CRT may even reverse NYHA class II heart failure. It is a minimally invasive procedure that does not require opening the chest to access the heart.

### Implantable Cardioverter-Defibrillators (ICDs)

An ICD is a device placed under the skin that can benefit many heart failure patients at high risk of sudden death from a rapid, irregular, disorganized heart rhythm. In fact, about half of all heart failure patients die suddenly from cardiac arrest. ICDs have been shown to be superior to anti-arrhythmic drugs in preventing sudden death. An

## Ventricular Assist Device

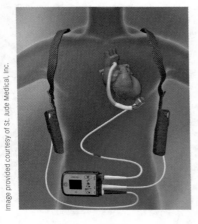

Image provided courtesy of St. Jude Medical, Inc.

A ventricular assist device (VAD) is a mechanical pump powered by a battery pack. It is inserted in the abdomen below the diaphragm and attached to the heart and the aorta. Blood flows from the left ventricle into the VAD and is propelled out to the body.

Miniaturized third-generation VADs, such as the HeartMate 3, have a single moving part that propels blood with a rotating turbine. The impeller is the device's only moving part. Suspended by magnets, it creates no friction and has no parts to wear out. Its biocompatible design reduces the risk of blood clots, infections, and strokes. As a result, it can be implanted permanently as an alternative to a human heart.

ICD can be combined with a biventricular pacemaker in a single device if a patient meets the criteria for both. CRT plus ICD has been shown to be particularly effective in women.

ICDs monitor heart rhythms. When ventricular tachycardia is detected, the ICD takes over by pacing the heart or delivering a shock that stops the arrhythmia and restores the heart's normal rhythm.

### Intra-Aortic Balloon Pumps

These mechanical devices are inserted into the aorta through an artery in the groin. A balloon is located at one end of a catheter, and the opposite end is connected to a computer console. The balloon pump is programmed to inflate and deflate in sync with the patient's heartbeat. When the heart contracts, the balloon collapses, easing the force required for ejecting blood from the left ventricle. When the heart relaxes, the balloon inflates, increasing the diastolic blood pressure in the aorta. Since coronary arteries receive most of their blood during diastole, inflation of the balloon improves coronary blood flow. Balloon pumps are used in the hospital's cardiac intensive care unit as temporary circulatory support in patients with acutely decompensated heart failure and cardiogenic shock.

### Ventricular Assist Devices

Perhaps the greatest change in heart failure treatment has been the advent of effective ventricular assist devices (VADs). Cleveland Clinic has one of the oldest and most active VAD programs in the country. It is one of the few working with a variety of FDA-approved VADs for patients with heart failure. This enables Cleveland Clinic surgeons to choose the device that best suits each patient's needs.

VADs support the heart in pumping oxygenated blood throughout the body. A battery power pack enables a VAD wearer to be out and about for several hours. This allows patients with advanced heart failure

to become more active and improve their health and fitness. VAD wearers waiting for a heart transplant are stronger and better able to withstand the stress of surgery when a donor heart becomes available.

VADs were developed as a "bridge to transplantation." They also are used as a permanent alternative in patients who are not eligible for heart transplantation. One-tenth to one-third of patients on a VAD and optimal medical therapy recover well enough to have the device removed. This means VADs also can be a "bridge to recovery."

The latest VADs are totally implantable and have a single moving part known as an impeller that propels blood with a rotating turbine. (It should not be confused with the temporary support device called Impella®.) It is suspended by magnets, creates no friction, and has no parts to wear out. It is highly biocompatible and resistant to wear and corrosion, making it ideal for permanent or long-term use. Its batteries can be recharged using household current.

Most VADs assist the left ventricle, the heart's main pumping chamber. For heart failure patients who also have a weakened right ventricle, some VADs are able to support either side of the heart. The latest VADs have success rates approaching that of heart transplantation, which remains a limited option due to the shortage of donor organs.

### Impella®

For patients with either systolic or diastolic heart failure requiring temporary support, Cleveland Clinic also uses a unique device known as the Impella®. A long tube, the Impella is inserted by catheter through the groin, into the heart, and across the aortic valve, where it rests in the left ventricle. As the heart pumps, a tiny turbine—about the size of a ballpoint-pen spring—inside the Impella helps pull blood out of the ventricle into the aorta, where it is pumped into the circulation.

## Total Artificial Hearts

In some patients with advanced heart failure, a heart transplant is the only option. But the wait for a donor heart can be long. In 2004, the FDA approved Syncardia's Total Artificial Heart® (TAH) for temporary use in patients eligible for heart transplantation and at risk for imminent death. To date, it has been used in more patients than any other total artificial heart. The TAH completely replaces a failing heart and is designed to restore normal blood pressure and cardiac output. This results in improved circulatory function that enables other organs jeopardized by inadequate blood supply to recover. The end result is that patients are better able to withstand and recover from their transplant.

## Coronary Artery Bypass Grafting

When CAD causes significant impairment of blood flow to the heart muscle, coronary artery bypass grafting (CABG) may be used to improve blood flow and relieve symptoms. Until 2011, no one knew whether the benefits of CABG would outweigh the risks in patients with heart failure and severe left ventricular dysfunction. The STICH trial shed light on the issue. This study randomized 1,212 patients to medical therapy alone or to medical therapy plus CABG and followed them for five years. CABG increased the risk of death for two years, after which time the number of deaths in patients on medical therapy alone became greater. During the five-year study period, CABG patients were less likely to die from cardiovascular causes than those on medications alone (28 percent versus 33 percent), or to require hospitalization for heart-related causes (58 percent versus 69 percent).

## Heart Transplantation

Heart transplantation remains the gold standard for treating end-stage heart failure, because it has proven to be the most effective treatment. More than half of all patients who have a heart transplant survive for more than 12 years. Unfortunately, the supply of donor hearts does not begin to meet demand: An estimated 20,000 to 70,000 people would benefit from a heart transplant, yet only about 2,000 a year receive one.

Heart transplantation is considered only when heart failure reaches NYHA class IV or ACC/AHA stage D, primarily due to the shortage of donor hearts. Patients are placed on the waiting list only after careful evaluation to determine their overall medical condition and whether alternative therapies might be useful. Screening determines whether the patient is likely to survive the operation and regain normal function.

Anyone being considered for a heart transplant must be capable of following a complex medical regimen and strict diet, quitting smoking, exercising regularly, and taking immunosuppressive drugs faithfully—a huge commitment. The presence of other serious medical conditions or psychological issues excludes some patients as transplant candidates, since medical compliance, emotional stability, and a strong support network of family and friends are critical to the operation's long-term success.

The biggest medical obstacle in heart transplantation is preventing the body from rejecting the donor heart. This is achieved through powerful immunosuppressive drugs, which must be taken for life. These drugs can cause serious side effects, so their dosing must be carefully adjusted and monitored to get the maximum protection with the fewest side effects.

Transplantation is not the answer to the widespread problem of heart failure. No one expects the supply of donor hearts ever to match the demand. Some patients are considered unsuitable candidates for transplantation. This has spurred researchers to concentrate on the development of better VADs to someday eliminate the need for a heart transplant.

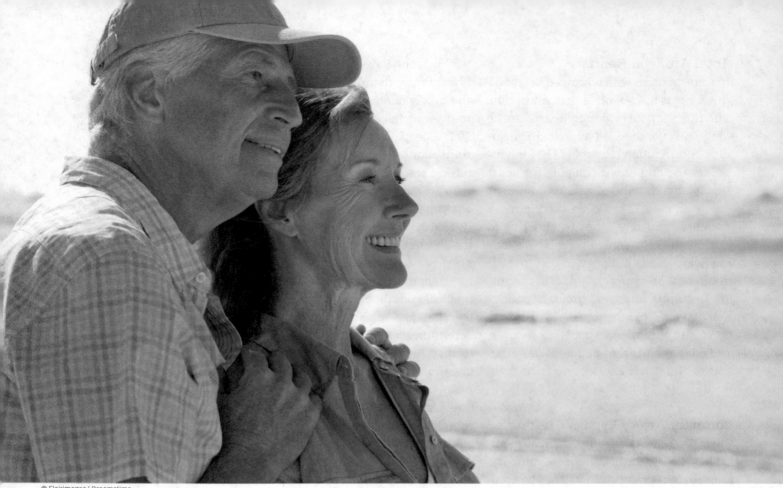

Every year, a higher percentage of people survive heart attacks and enjoy an extended quality of life after the event. Working with your doctor is the key.

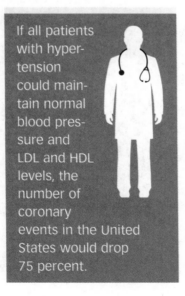

If all patients with hypertension could maintain normal blood pressure and LDL and HDL levels, the number of coronary events in the United States would drop 75 percent.

## 8 Looking Ahead to A Longer, Better Life

Advances in the prevention and treatment of CAD are taking place with astounding speed. We have become more adept at protecting the heart by reducing or eliminating risk factors and preventing debilitating or fatal heart attacks or heart failure. Treatment methods are becoming more patient friendly, which helps ensure compliance. And thanks to new medications, heart disease is doing less permanent damage. Recuperation and recovery time have been greatly reduced, and patients are resuming an active lifestyle after a heart attack or interventional therapy more quickly than ever before.

Fortunately, a growing number of people are taking a proactive role in preventing heart disease by exercising more and eating better. We have learned that a heart-healthy diet not only helps prevent CAD, but also makes us feel better and improves our quality of life.

### On the Horizon

If you have CAD, your attitude toward your disease and your doctor's approach to managing it are likely to change over the next few years as more information about preventing and treating CAD becomes available. You can expect to see:

- Medications that will delay or prevent the need for more extensive (and expensive) treatment.
- Medications that can reverse CAD.
- Medications that can stop or dramatically limit the damage from a heart attack.
- A more personalized approach using genetics to determine CAD risk and to predict the usefulness of certain medications in a given patient.
- Increasing emphasis placed on quality of life and the role of psychosocial factors in heart disease.

The search for novel approaches to prevent and treat CAD and its complications will continue.

While new approaches are being tested in clinical trials, science is looking at different ways to improve heart surgery, reduce damage from heart attack, and, ultimately, prevent CAD. Some of these new approaches discussed in this section will be refined until researchers are satisfied that they offer a better, more agreeable or less-expensive way of treating heart disease. Developments to watch include:

### Improving Medication Adherence

Why heart patients don't take their medications faithfully or consistently is not always clear. The worst offenders are those at highest risk, including smokers and patients with diabetes and heart failure. Consistent use of evidence-based heart medications such as beta-blockers, aspirin, and statins is known to increase the chance of long-term survival.

According to the American College of Cardiology, at least 2 million cardiovascular events per year could be avoided if high blood pressure and high cholesterol were controlled. If all patients with hypertension would maintain normal blood pressure and LDL and HDL levels, the number of coronary events in the United States would drop 75 percent. Yet compliance with statins, which are known to have strongly cardioprotective effects, is very poor: A very high percentage of patients taking statins stop taking the medication after about two years, increasing their risk for heart attack. Researchers are trying various ways to increase compliance, including developing medications that can be taken once or twice a year—at least less often than daily.

### Reducing Systemic Inflammation to Prevent CAD

Researchers have long felt that the beneficial effect of statins is partly due to their anti-inflammatory properties, in addition to their LDL-lowering capability. This theory was successfully tested in the Canakinumab Anti-inflammatory Thrombosis Outcome Study (CANTOS). Canakinumab is a monoclonal antibody that reduces inflammation, but has no effect on cholesterol or other blood lipids.

In this trial of 10,000 patients with prior heart attack and systemic inflammation (as gauged by elevated levels of C-reactive protein), those given canakinumab had 15 percent fewer heart attacks and strokes than those given placebo. Fewer events occurred even in patients on optimal statin therapy. Canakinumab also reduced the need for revascularization about 30 percent over a four-year period.

CANTOS revealed that fighting inflammation is an exciting new strategy for reducing the impact of CAD and deaths caused by the disease. As a result, we can expect to see a variety of inflammation-fighting medications tested in the near future—even as you are reading this report. These medications may include the TNF-alpha inhibitors etanercept (Embrel®), adalimumab (Humira®), and infliximab (Remicade®), as well as methotrexate (Rheumatrex®, Trexall®) and other biologics used in rheumatoid arthritis, inflammatory bowel disease, psoriasis, lupus, and celiac disease. The presence of these chronic inflammatory diseases greatly increases the likelihood of developing CAD and having a heart attack, and it is hoped the anti-inflammatory medications used to treat them will reduce the amount of plaque deposited in artery walls.

### Tackling Diastolic Heart Failure

Medication and devices for heart failure are primarily directed at patients with systolic heart failure, also known as heart failure with reduced ejection fraction (HFrRF). In this form of heart failure, the left ventricle—the heart's primary pumping chamber—does not contract strongly enough to eject a sufficient amount of blood into the circulation. The ejection fraction, or amount of blood ejected with each squeeze, drops.

There is a second form of heart failure called diastolic heart failure, also called heart failure with preserved ejection fraction (HFpEF). In these patients, the heart pumps well, but its walls become stiff and unable to expand properly. The heart fails to fill with blood at normal pressures, and blood backs up in the lungs and circulation, causing shortness of breath and swelling. Medications to reduce these pressures and their associated symptoms have not been successful.

The inter-atrial shunt device (IASD) appears to do what medications cannot. The IASD creates an opening between the right and left sides of the heart, so that blood can flow from the high-pressure left atrium to the low-pressure right atrium. This lowers the pressure in the left atrium and lungs. In the first IASD study, patients who received the device showed lasting improvements in NYHA class and quality of life and were able to walk further without fatigue. Cleveland Clinic will be participating in future clinical trials of this device.

## Using Stem Cells to Repair the Heart

The potential to regenerate heart muscle using stem cells is an intriguing area of research. Many clinical trials are ongoing, but approval by the U.S. Food & Drug Administration is years away.

Among the issues yet to be determined are the type of stem cell that works best, how the cells should be given to a patient, and how many cells are needed to produce effective results. Unfortunately, there is too much variety in stem cell trials conducted to date to answer these questions. This is what we know so far about stem-cell therapy:

- In the United States, you must be in a clinical trial to receive stem cell therapy.
- Bone marrow-derived mononuclear stem cells (BMMS) are safe and do not produce a reaction from the immune system that requires immunosuppressant drugs. Mesenchymal stem cells (MSCs) also may be safe, but the jury is still out. Skeletal myoblasts are no longer used, because they cause potentially deadly arrhythmias.
- Stem cells taken from younger people are more robust than those taken from older individuals.
- Stem cells taken from the patient and returned to the patient (autogenic cells) are safe. Stem cells taken from another person (allogenic) also can be safely used, which gives older patients hope for a better outcome.
- Stem cells can be effective when delivered directly into the heart muscle or into a coronary artery.
- After being injected, stem cells may not take root and populate. Instead, they may release substances that recruit the host tissue to repair the damage. The stem cells themselves disappear after several weeks, but their beneficial effect may last as long as six months.
- When stem cells cause a measurable improvement in the heart—for example, by minimizing scar tissue, increasing blood flow to the heart muscle, or improving ejection fraction—heart function may not noticeably improve. When significant improvement in heart function does occur, it is usually in the form of improved ejection fraction.

Large, well-designed studies that are now underway will increase our understanding of whether the effects of stem-cell therapy can decrease symptoms of diseases such as heart failure and improve survival.

Researchers have found a way to isolate the basic cellular framework of the heart (its matrix) and use stem cells to grow heart tissue on it. However, they have not yet determined whether the new tissue is strong enough to pump blood through the body, or how long it might last. Whether stem cells are a viable option for patients with CAD may not be known for decades.

## Using Stem Cells to Reverse Stroke Damage

Cleveland Clinic researchers are participating in a multicenter study to determine whether calming the body's immune response to stroke can limit or reverse permanent damage to the brain. Most stroke research projects of this type have focused on implanting stem cells directly into the brain, where it is hoped they will create new brain tissue to replace that damaged by stroke. Instead, this new study is infusing stem cells into the bloodstream, with the hope they will prevent the immune system from overreacting and harming the brain. To date, those who have been infused have had less disability than expected at 90 days. The researchers feel the technique is unlikely to prevent or totally reverse stroke damage, but may cut damage at least in half.

## Using Gene Therapy to Grow New Blood Vessels

By manipulating genes, researchers have found that the heart can grow tiny new blood vessels in a process known as angiogenesis. These vessels are much smaller than normal vessels and will not restore normal blood flow, but they appear able to bring long-awaited relief from angina.

Much research is concentrating on gene therapy with a protein called vascular endothelial growth factor (VEGF), but other proteins such as platelet-derived endothelial cell growth factor (PD-ECGF) also are being considered. Cleveland Clinic cardiologists say VEGF is most effective when injected directly into the heart muscle during open-heart surgery. It is hoped VEGF may become an option for patients who have no other treatment choice, and it may be used to augment bypass surgery.

## Predicting Who Will Get CAD

How can someone who eats cholesterol-laden foods, never exercises, and smokes two packs of cigarettes a day avoid a heart attack, while someone else who behaves

**NEW FINDING**

### Use Exercise to Combat the Heart Risk You Inherit

As physical fitness and strength increase, the risk of heart attack and stroke falls, as does the risk of atrial fibrillation. In one large study, more than 500,000 participants in a U.K. database were divided into three levels (standard deviations, or SD) of physical activity, grip strength, and cardiorespiratory fitness. Each SD of fitness lowered the risk of coronary artery disease (CAD) 25 percent, atrial fibrillation 39 percent and cardiovascular events 31 percent. Each SD in grip strength lowered the risk in all three categories 12 to 13 percent. Risk of death also was greatly diminished with each SD increase in fitness and grip strength. The study also showed that the fitter, stronger participants had lower risks of cardiovascular events and atrial fibrillation in every genetic risk category. Those considered to be at high risk for heart attack or stroke, but who were the most physically fit, had a 49 percent lower risk of coronary artery disease and 60 percent lower risk of atrial fibrillation than their peers. Those with a strong grip were 31 percent less likely to develop CAD and 39 percent less likely to develop atrial fibrillation than others with the same genetic risk who were less fit. This suggests that the higher your genetic risk, the greater the benefit you will derive from increasing your cardiorespiratory fitness and muscle strength.

*Circulation,* April 9, 2018

the same way dies from one? Whether you develop CAD depends on your behavior and your family history. There is nothing you can do about the genes you have, but there may be steps you can take to reduce your risk of getting CAD if you inherit these genes (see "Use Exercise to Combat the Heart Risk You Inherit").

Scientists have been cataloging genes of people who are healthy and those who have been stricken with any number of different diseases, including CAD. To date, 17 gene variants that appear only in, or mostly in, people who develop CAD have been identified. There are several benefits to this concept.

- If the protein product of the gene is involved in causing the disease, drug companies may be able to create a drug that inhibits this disease-causing activity.

- You would be able to be screened to see if you carry that gene. If you do, you would be able to modify your lifestyle earlier to delay, and perhaps even prevent, the onset of symptoms.

- Finally, if you know what gene causes heart disease, it might become possible to silence it with gene therapy.

## Printing New Valves and Hearts

It sounds like science fiction, but researchers at Cleveland Clinic and other research centers are printing organs on 3-D printers stocked not with paper, but with viable human tissue. To date, ears, bones, and muscles have been created and successfully implanted in animals. Cleveland Clinic pediatric heart surgeons have used 3-D printers to replicate complex heart deformities prior to corrective surgery. In the near future, it may be possible to order a heart valve or blood vessel to be printed to a patient's specifications.

## A Last Word...

As you have learned, the prevention and treatment of CAD are life-and-death issues. Cardiologists and surgeons have more tools at their disposal than ever before to help CAD patients live longer and with a better quality of life. But whether you can manage your risk factors and avoid CAD, or thrive after heart surgery or revascularization, is up to you (see "Get a Flu Shot!"). You may have a great team of health-care providers to work with, but your choices and behaviors will ultimately dictate whether you and your team succeed.

If you can work with a physician and medical center with extensive experience and expertise in heart care—preferably one that conducts research and uses a team approach to care—it will increase your chance of having a successful outcome. Your doctor will be more likely to use the newest medications and the latest techniques for your care. It also may give you access to clinical trials, if standard procedures do not work for you.

Keep on doing what you are doing now—educating yourself about the latest in cardiovascular care. During your next appointment, discuss what you've learned from reading this Special Report with your physician. Follow his or her recommendations closely, and speak up about any concerns or questions you may have. Remember that there are no shortcuts when it comes to the health of your heart. It may take time to arrive at the best treatment plan for you. But if you are willing to make the necessary lifestyle adjustments and work in tandem with your physician, you stand the best chance of living a longer and better life.

**If you have CAD, you may hear many of the terms used in this report, but not always understand what they mean. This glossary is designed to help you. If you want more information on any term, ask your doctor.**

**acute coronary syndrome (ACS):** The presence of unstable angina, a non-ST-segment elevation myocardial infarction (NSTEMI), or an ST-segment elevation myocardial infarction (STEMI).

**angina (also called angina pectoris):** Discomfort or pain in the chest that occurs when fatty plaques that narrow coronary arteries interfere with blood supply to the heart muscle.

**angiogram:** A moving x-ray image of blood flowing through coronary arteries.

**angioplasty:** A treatment in which a special catheter with an inflatable balloon at its tip is threaded into a narrowing area of a coronary artery caused by plaque buildup.

**antiarrhythmics:** Drugs that control the heart's rhythm.

**anticoagulants:** Drugs that prevent blood from clotting.

**antiplatelet agents:** Drugs that inhibit the activation of platelets and, in so doing, help prevent blood from clotting; they include aspirin and clopidogrel (Plavix®), ticagrelor (Brilinta®), and prasugrel (Effient®).

**aorta:** The large, main artery exiting the heart. All blood pumped out of the left ventricle travels through the aorta on its way to other parts of the body.

**arrhythmias:** Abnormal heart rhythms.

**artery:** Blood vessel that carries oxygenated blood from the heart to the organs and tissues.

**atherosclerosis:** Deposits of fatty substances, cholesterol, calcium and fibrin (the protein that forms a blood clot) in the arteries, which can block blood flow.

**atrium (pl. atria):** An upper chamber of the heart that receives blood from the veins.

**blood clot (thrombus):** A clot forms when clotting factors in the blood cause it to coagulate or become a jelly-like mass. When a blood clot forms inside a blood vessel (a thrombus), it can dislodge, travel through the bloodstream, and become trapped, causing a heart attack or stroke.

**calcification:** A process in which tissue becomes hardened due to deposits of calcium. Calcification of blood vessels plays a role in the development of atherosclerosis.

**cardiac catheterization:** An imaging procedure that involves inserting a catheter into a blood vessel in the arm or leg, and guiding it to the heart with the aid of x-ray movies. Contrast dye injected through the catheter allows the coronary arteries to be seen (coronary angiography).

**catheter:** A long, thin tube that is inserted into the arteries or veins for diagnostic or therapeutic purposes. Cardiologists can measure pressures, inject contrast dye and drugs, insert tools for measurements (See IVUS), and insert stents through catheters.

**cholesterol:** A waxy, fat-like substance found in foods of animal origin and synthesized by the body. It is used for many of the body's processes, including hormone production. In large amounts in the blood, cholesterol can clog arteries.

**contrast agent:** An iodine-containing dye that is denser than the surrounding heart tissue. When it is mixed with the blood, the blood vessels can be seen with x-rays, as during coronary angiography.

**coronary angiography:** A procedure using a contrast agent and moving x-rays to show blood flow through coronary arteries. Selective coronary angiography, in which a catheter is inserted into the mouth of one of the coronary arteries (left or right) followed by the injection of dye helped pave the way for coronary artery bypass surgery and stenting.

**coronary artery bypass grafting (CABG):** A surgical procedure in which a vein or an artery is taken from another part of your body and sewn to your heart to create a new conduit for blood to flow around (bypass) a blocked coronary artery.

**coronary artery disease (CAD):** A condition caused by the buildup of fatty plaques in the artery walls, which narrows the blood vessels and prevents enough oxygen from reaching the heart. CAD is the most common type of heart disease.

**diabetes:** A condition in which the body does not produce or properly use the hormone insulin, which is needed to convert sugar, starches, and other food into energy.

**diastolic pressure:** The blood pressure in the arteries when the heart is filling with blood. It is the lower of two blood pressure measurements. For example, in a blood pressure reading of 120/80 mmHg, 80 is the diastolic pressure.

**diuretics:** Drugs that remove excess fluid from the tissues and bloodstream, lessen edema (swelling).

**dyslipidemia:** Abnormal levels of lipids (fat-soluble molecules) in the blood.

**echocardiogram:** An imaging procedure that creates a moving picture of the heart's valves and chambers using high-frequency sound waves emanating from a device placed on the chest or guided into the esophagus behind the heart. Echocardiography is used to evaluate blood flow through the heart's valves.

**edema:** Swelling due to water retention.

**ejection fraction:** The percentage of blood in the ventricles pumped out with each beat. A normal ejection fraction is 55 to 65 percent. The lower the percentage, the more advanced the heart failure.

**endothelium:** The thin layer of cells that lines the inside of blood vessels.

**epicardium:** The outermost layer of the heart, which contains the coronary arteries and veins.

**exercise stress test:** A test used to provide information about how the heart responds to stress. It usually involves walking on a treadmill or pedaling a stationary bike at increasing levels of difficulty, while the electrocardiogram, heart rate, and blood pressure are monitored.

**heart attack:** Injury or death of some heart muscle, usually caused by a blood clot in the heart.

**heart failure (congestive heart failure, CHF):** A chronic, progressive disease in which the heart muscle weakens and can no longer pump blood well enough to meet the body's needs.

**heart-lung machine:** A machine that performs the task of pumping blood and providing oxygen to the blood during open-heart surgery, also known as cardiopulmonary bypass.

**high-density lipoprotein (HDL) cholesterol:** A type of lipoprotein particle that carries "bad" (LDL) cholesterol to the liver for excretion. HDL-C is "good" cholesterol and reduces cholesterol buildup in the arteries.

**hypertension:** High blood pressure.

**hyperkalemia:** Elevated potassium levels.

**inotropic agent:** A type of drug that stimulates the heart to contract.

**interventional cardiology:** A clinical field that involves using devices such as catheters inserted into the arteries or veins for diagnostic and therapeutic purposes.

**intravascular ultrasound (IVUS):** A technique used during left heart catheterization that allows interventional cardiologists to accurately measure the coronary artery diameter and the components of its wall (normal, soft plaque, calcified plaque) and to determine whether a stent is fully expanded inside the vessel.

**ischemia:** Pronounced "iss-KEE-mee-uh," it is a deficiency in blood flow to a tissue or organ resulting in insufficient oxygen delivery to the cells. Angina occurs due to ischemia of the heart muscle tissue.

**left ventricular assist device (LVAD):** An implanted mechanical device that pumps blood directly to assist a failing heart.

**lipid:** A term encompassing many kinds of fat-soluble molecules, including cholesterol, triglycerides, and free fatty acids.

**lipoprotein:** A specialized, microscopic, spherical particle in the blood composed of protein and lipids. Its role is to move lipids from one part of the body to another.

**low-density lipoprotein (LDL) cholesterol:** A type of lipoprotein particle that carries cholesterol to the tissues, where it can build up and lead to heart disease, from the liver. LDL-C is "bad" cholesterol.

**magnetic resonance imaging (MRI):** An imaging technique that uses magnetic fields instead of x-rays to create images of internal structures in the body, including the brain, heart, and other organs.

**metabolic syndrome:** Having three or more of the following conditions: high triglycerides, low HDL cholesterol, high blood pressure, elevated blood glucose, and a large waist circumference.

**myocardial infarction (MI):** The medical term for a heart attack.

**myocardial perfusion:** The amount of blood flowing through the heart muscle; a myocardial perfusion imaging test, also called a nuclear stress test, shows how much blood is reaching the heart and how strongly the heart muscle is pumping.

**myocardium:** The heart muscle.

**NSTEMI (non-ST-segment elevation myocardial infarction):** A type of mild heart attack in which a portion (the ST-segment) of the line produced during an electrocardiogram test is not elevated.

**pacemaker:** An electronic device that is implanted under the skin and sends electrical impulses to the heart muscle to maintain a desired heart rate.

**percutaneous coronary intervention (PCI):** Any procedure performed by cardiologists inside the coronary arteries to improve blood flow, including angioplasty, stenting, rotablation, and other techniques.

**plaque:** Fatty deposits that form on the inside surface of arteries that are characteristic of atherosclerosis.

**platelets:** Small cells that circulate in the blood and help form blood clots.

**pulse rate:** The number of heartbeats per minute. The resting pulse rate for an average adult is between 60 and 80 beats per minute (BPM).

**remodeling:** Changes in the size, shape, and function of the heart and blood vessels.

**restenosis:** Recurrent development of atherosclerosis at the same location, or narrowing of the blood vessel recurring at the same location where stenting or balloon angioplasty has been performed.

**revascularization:** Procedures, such as coronary artery bypass grafting, balloon angioplasty or stenting, that restore or increase blood flow through a coronary artery.

**septum:** The wall between the two ventricles.

**STEMI (ST-segment elevation myocardial infarction):** A major heart attack in which the ST-segment of the electrocardiogram (ECG) is elevated due to complete blockage of a coronary artery.

**stenosis:** A narrowing of a blood vessel.

**stent:** A small, flexible tube made of metal mesh that can be inserted into arteries to expand narrow openings.

**sudden cardiac death:** Death that occurs when the heart abruptly stops pumping, most commonly from a disturbance in the heart's electrical system.

**systolic pressure:** The pressure of the blood in the arteries when the heart contracts. It is the higher of two blood pressure measurements. In a blood pressure reading of 120/80 mmHg, 120 is the systolic pressure.

**thrombosis:** The formation of a clot inside a blood vessel or stent, which rapidly leads to a heart attack.

**vein:** A blood vessel that carries deoxygenated blood back toward the heart.

**ventricle:** A thick, muscular chamber of the heart that pumps blood from the heart into the arteries

**American College of Cardiology**
www.acc.org
Resource@acc.org
800-253-4636, Ext. 5603
2400 N. St., NW
Washington, DC 20037

**American Heart Association**
www.heart.org
800-242-8721
7272 Greenville Ave.
Dallas, TX 75231

**American Society of Transplantation**
www.myast.org
856-439-9986
1120 Route 73, Suite 200
Mt. Laurel, NJ 08054

**Heart Failure Society of America**
www.hfsa.org
info@hfsa.org
301-312-8635
9211 Corporate Blvd., Suite 270
Bethesda, MD 20850

**National Heart, Lung and Blood Institute**
www.nhlbi.nih.gov/health
301-496-4000

**WomenHeart: The National Coalition for Women with Heart Disease**
www.womenheart.org
mail@womenheart.org
202-728-7199
1100 17th St., NW, Suite 500
Washington, DC 20036

**Cleveland Clinic Sydell and Arnold Miller Family Heart and Vascular Institute**
www.myclevelandclinic.org/services/heart
9500 Euclid Ave.
Cleveland, OH 44195

For more information, call the Heart and Vascular Nurse at 866-289-6911 (toll free).

For an appointment with a cardiologist or cardiac surgeon, call 800-659-7822 (toll free).

## IF YOU ARE HAVING ANY OF THESE SYMPTOMS:

### CALL YOUR DOCTOR

- Weight gain of more than three pounds in one day or five pounds in one week
- Swelling in your ankles, legs, or abdomen that has become worse
- Shortness of breath that has become worse, especially if you awaken short of breath
- Extreme fatigue or decreased activity tolerance
- A respiratory infection or cough that has become worse
- Fast heart rate (above 100 beats per minute)
- Episodes of chest pain or discomfort with exertion that are relieved with rest
- Difficulty breathing with normal activities or at rest
- Severe dizziness, lightheadedness, or fainting
- Nausea or poor appetite

### CALL 911

**Call 911 if you are experiencing any of the symptoms of a heart attack:**

- New chest pain or discomfort that is severe, unexpected, and accompanied by shortness of breath, sweating, nausea, or weakness, and/or is unrelieved by nitroglycerin
- Fast, sustained heart rate (more than 120 beats per minute), especially if you are short of breath, dizzy, or lightheaded
- Shortness of breath that is not relieved by rest
- Sudden weakness or paralysis in your arms or legs
- Loss of consciousness

### IN CASE OF EMERGENCY

FILL IN THESE DETAILS AND LEAVE THEM IN A PROMINENT PLACE (FOR EXAMPLE, TAPED TO THE REFRIGERATOR) FOR FAMILY, FRIENDS, AND PARAMEDICS IN CASE OF EMERGENCY.

| MY DATE OF BIRTH AND AGE: | MY DOCTOR'S NAME AND ADDRESS: | MY PHARMACY (NAME, PHONE, ADDRESS): |
|---|---|---|
| MY ADDRESS: | | |
| MY PHONE NUMBER: | MY DOCTOR'S PHONE NUMBER: | MY MEDICATIONS (INCLUDE DOSAGE): |
| MY INSURANCE INFORMATION: | NAME AND ADDRESS OF HOSPITAL NEAREST TO ME: | |